Preface

The General Dental Council Recommendations concerning the dental curriculum indicate that dental students should be able to understand human disease as far as it is relevant to the practice of dentistry. Indeed, modern dental practice has an increasingly important basis in medicine and surgery, particularly with the rising elderly population and numbers of patients suffering various syste[illegible] disorders such as the immunological diseases. In addition, th[illegible]g complexity of operative dental, oral and maxillofacial [illegible]d oral medicine and pathology warrants a substantial [illegible] of medical matters as is recognized in the MFDS RCS [illegible]. We are not aware of any other colour illustrated text [illegible]

[illegible] therefore is intended to help trainees of *all* dental [illegible]ties, postgraduates and practitioners. In particular, it hopefully provides the reader with an awareness of the major clinical features [illegible]dical and surgical disorders, of the extraoral fe[illegible]orders with prominent oral features, and of those [illegible]s that influence dental management.

In view of space restrictions, the book cannot be completely comprehensive, and does not cover pharmacological or psychological medicine, parasitic, exotic or tropical diseases, or obstetric[illegible] and gynaecology. More specialized texts should be consulte[illegible] where additional detail is sought.

We would like to acknowledge the help of Frances Scully for Figure 29, Simon Porter for Figure 17, Dr Mohamed Elkabir for Figure 65, Connie Blake for Figure 66 and Professor Alan Harrison (University of Bristol) for providing Figures 147 and 148, and the curator of the museum at Guy's Hospital. We are indebted to Martin Dunitz Ltd. for permission to reproduce Figures 7 and 152 from *Colour Atlas of Oral Disease* (Scully, C., Flint, S., Porter, S. R. Dunitz: London, 1996).

S. R. P.
1999 C. S.
P. W.
M. G.

Contents

1 / Infectious disease

Herpes simplex

Aetiology Herpes simplex viruses (HSV) types 1 (infections mainly oral and above the waist) and 2 (mainly genital as a sexually transmitted disease).

Pathology Virus spreads in secretions and infects epithelium, secondarily spreading to sensory neurones where it remains latent.

Clinical features Incubation 3–7 days.

Herpetic stomatitis: pyrexia, mouth ulcers (Fig. 1), gingival swelling and cervical lymphadenopathy.

Genital and ano-rectal herpes: typically in an adult with blisters and sores.

Investigations Electron-microscopy or immunostaining of vesicle fluid, culture, polymerase chain reaction (PCR) or serology.

Management Symptomatic; aciclovir mainly for the immunocompromised.

Complications *Herpes labialis:* reactivation causes herpes on lips (cold sores, Fig. 3) or other mucocutaneous junctions. Papules are followed by blisters then pustules. Treatment is with penciclovir cream.

Chickenpox

Aetiology Varicella zoster virus (VZV).

Pathology Transmission is by droplets.

Clinical features Incubation 11–20 days followed by fever and centripetal rash (Fig. 2). Pruritic macules progress to papules, vesicles, then pustules.

Investigations Not usually required.

Management Symptomatic; aciclovir for the immunocompromised.

Prevention Zoster immune globulin may protect high-risk contacts, e.g. the immunocompromised.

Complications Herpes zoster (see p. 3).

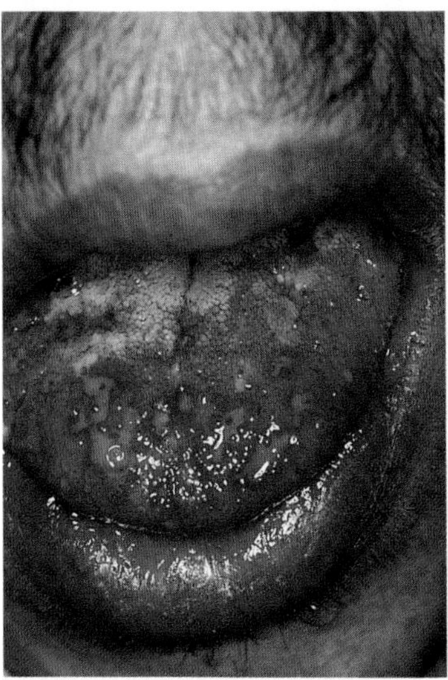

Fig. 1 Multiple ragged oral ulceration in primary HSV infection.

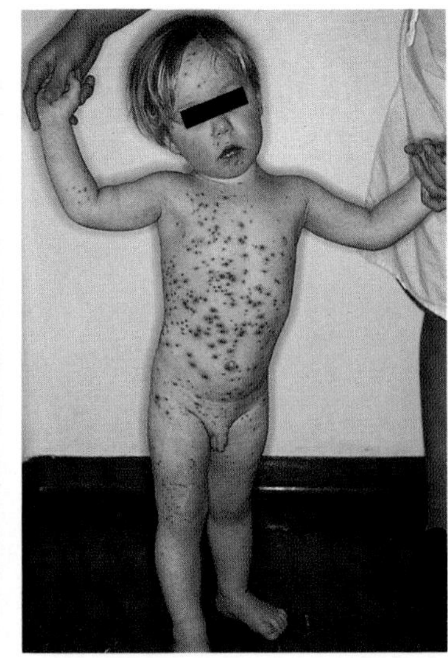

Fig. 2 Chickenpox: note the centripetal distribution of the rash.

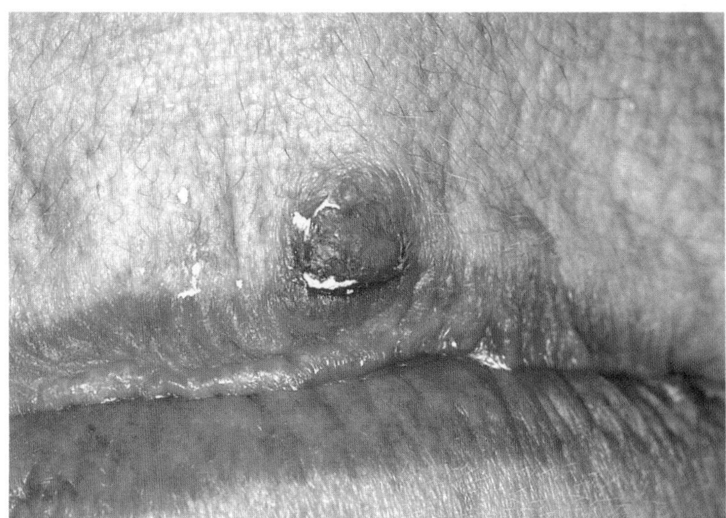

Fig. 3 Herpes labialis.

Herpes zoster (Shingles)

Aetiology

Reactivation of VZV typically at a late age or with immune suppression.

Clinical features

Pain and rash (Figs 4 & 5) in affected mucosa and dermatome—usually thoracolumbar or facial.

Management

Systemic aciclovir. Eye care if appropriate.

Infectious mononucleosis (glandular fever)

Glandular fever is the association of fever, sore throat and generalized lymphadenopathy seen mainly in Epstein–Barr virus, cytomegalovirus, HIV, human herpesvirus 6 (HHV-6) or toxoplasma infection.

Aetiology

Epstein–Barr virus (EBV).

Pathology

Virus presumably spreads by saliva, with infection of oropharyngeal epithelium and B lymphocytes.

Clinical features

Fever, sore throat, faucial oedema (Fig. 6) and generalized lymphadenopathy. Rarely, there is upper respiratory obstruction, possibly life threatening.

Investigations

- Blood film (abnormal lymphocytosis).
- Heterophile antibody test (Monospot or Paul–Bunnell test usually positive).
- Anti-EBV antibodies.

Management

Symptomatic.

Papillomavirus infections

Aetiology

There are over 75 human papillomaviruses (HPV).

Pathology and clinical features

HPV are probably transmitted by touch, are epitheliotrophic and usually cause benign warty lesions on skin and mucosae (Fig. 7).

Investigations

Histology is occasionally valuable.

Management

- Salicylate or podophyllum ointments.
- Surgical removal—cryotherapy, laser or excision.

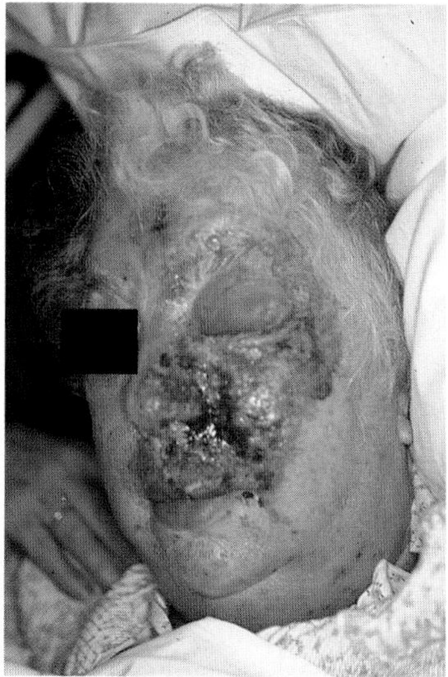

Fig. 4 Shingles of left maxillary division of trigeminal nerve.

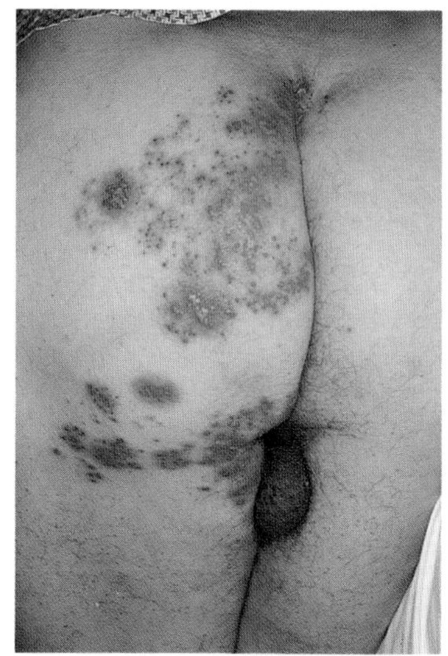

Fig. 5 Shingles of sacral nerve roots: bladder dysfunction may be present.

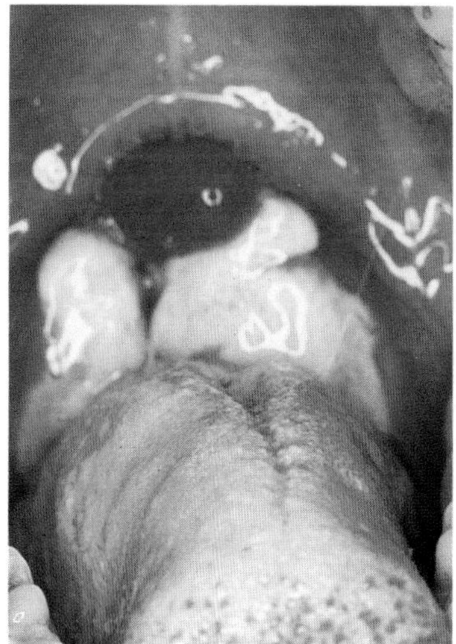

Fig. 6 Faucial oedema and slough in glandular fever.

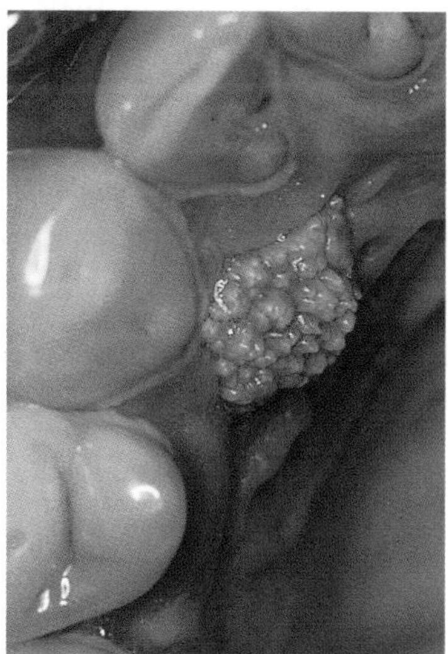

Fig. 7 Papillomatous oral lesion of HPV infection.

HIV infection

Aetiology

Human immunodeficiency viruses (HIV).

Pathology

Transmitted in blood or by sexual contact. HIV infects CD4 + T lymphocytes and brain glial cells.

Clinical features

Glandular fever-like illness about 6 weeks after infection but clinical manifestations of acquired immune deficiency syndrome (AIDS, Fig. 8) follow up to 15 years later. These include:

- *opportunistic infections*—especially *Pneumocystis carinii* pneumonia, candidosis (Fig. 9), herpesvirus infections, and tuberculosis
- *malignant neoplasms*—especially Kaposi's sarcoma (Fig. 10) and lymphomas
- *autoimmune disease*—e.g. thrombocytopenic purpura.

Oral manifestations are common and include candidosis, oral hairy leukoplakia (EBV infection) (Fig. 11) and Kaposi's sarcoma (Human herpesvirus 8 infection).

Investigations

Serology or viral culture is definitive.

Management and prevention

Nucleoside analogues, non-nucleoside reverse transcriptase inhibitors and protease inhibitors. Treat infections or neoplasms. Health education.

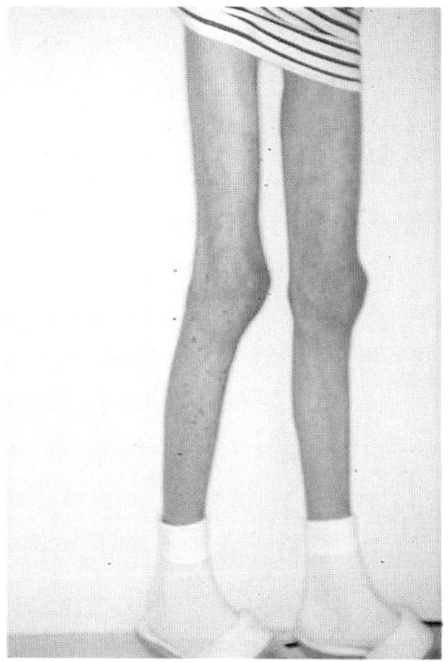

Fig. 8 Profound wasting in AIDS: 'Slim disease'.

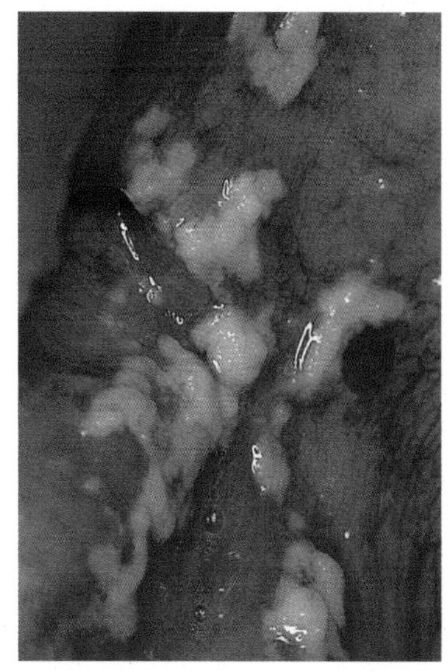

Fig. 9 Severe candidal infection in HIV disease.

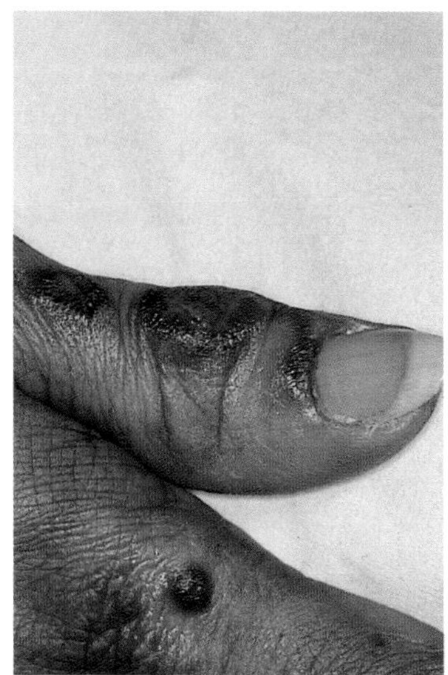

Fig. 10 Kaposi's sarcoma in HIV disease.

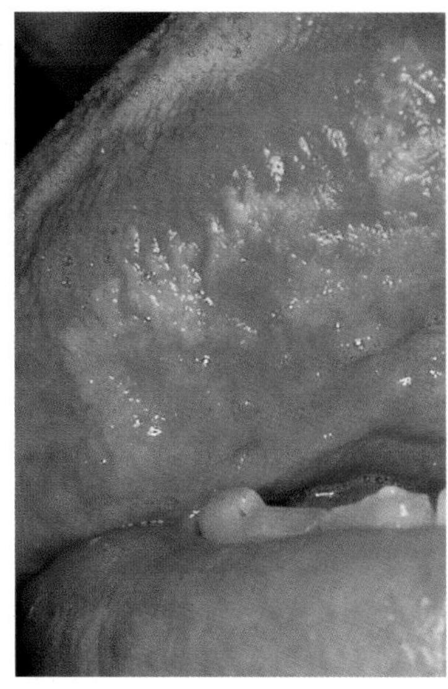

Fig. 11 Oral hairy leukoplakia.

Mumps

Aetiology Mumps virus. Dissemination by droplets.

Clinical features Incubation 2–3 weeks followed by pyrexia, malaise, headache and painful salivary gland swellings (Fig. 12), pancreatic, ovarian and testicular involvement can occur.

Investigations Viral culture; serum antibody levels; amylase (raised).

Management and prevention Supportive care. Vaccinate at 1 year (mumps, measles, rubella (MMR) vaccine).

Measles

Aetiology Measles virus spread by droplets.

Clinical features Incubation 7–10 days followed by: fever, Koplik's spots (white papules in buccal mucosa, Fig. 13) and a maculopapular rash (Fig. 14).

Management and prevention Symptomatic. Vaccinate at 1 year (MMR vaccine).

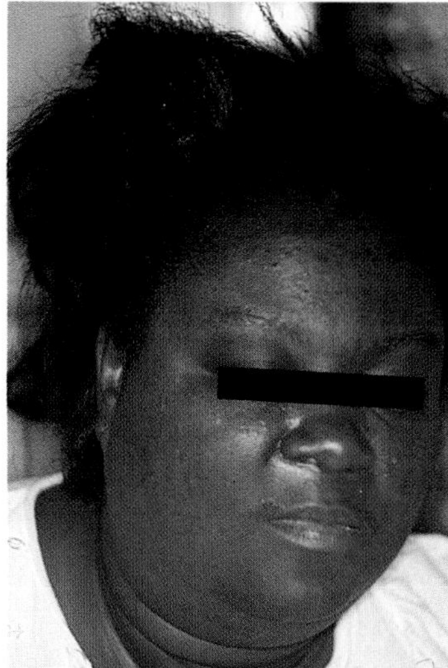

Fig. 12 Parotid enlargement in mumps.

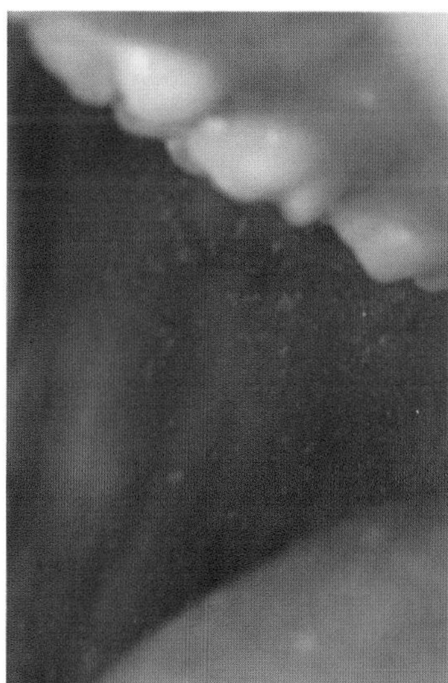

Fig. 13 Koplik's spots in measles.

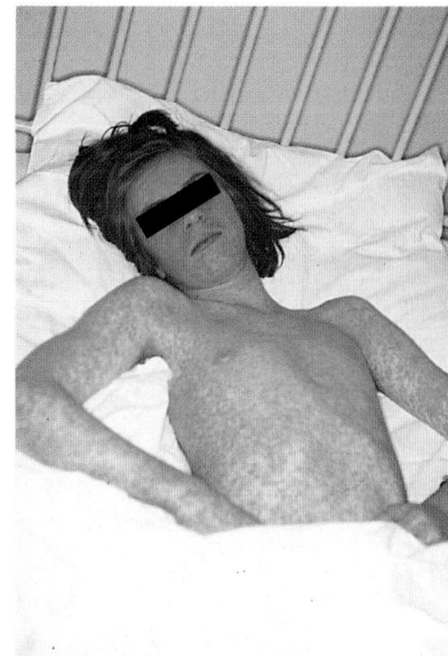

Fig. 14 Rash of measles.

Rubella (German measles)

Aetiology Rubella virus, spread by droplets.

Clinical features Incubation 14–21 days followed by a mild, pink macular rash (Fig. 15), fever and lymphadenopathy (often suboccipital).

Management Symptomatic.

Congenital rubella
Rubella infection of a non-immune pregnant woman may damage fetal hearing, eyes, brain and heart.

Prevention Vaccinate at 1 year (MMR vaccine).

Influenza

Aetiology Influenza virus—mainly types A and B. Droplet spread.

Clinical features Incubation 2 days followed by fever, myalgia, headache and malaise.

Management Symptomatic; with or without amantadine.

Prevention Vaccines protect against some strains.

Poliomyelitis

Aetiology Poliomyelitis virus, disseminated by ingestion.

Clinical features Incubation 3–30 days. Infection is mostly asymptomatic, but a minority have respiratory or gastrointestinal upset or headache, muscle pain and stiffness. Later flaccid paralysis develops (Fig. 16). Involvement of vital centres can lead to respiratory paralysis and death.

Management Supportive. Tracheostomy may be needed for prolonged respiratory support.

Prevention Vaccination. Shortly destined for worldwide eradication.

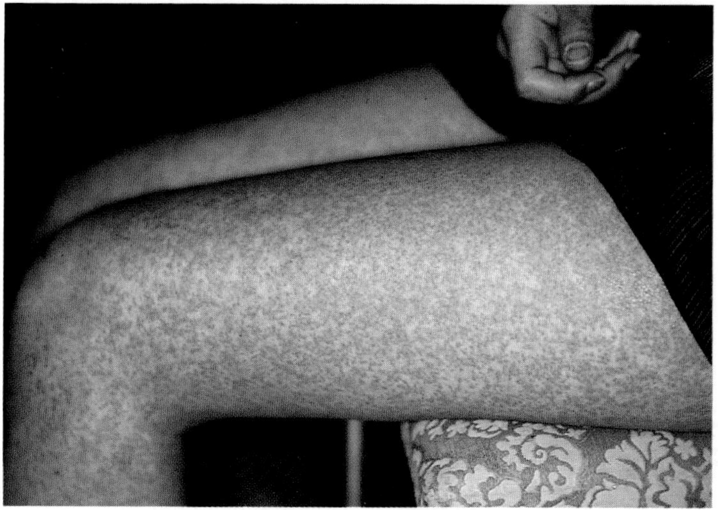

Fig. 15 Rash of rubella. In this patient the rash is particularly extensive and florid.

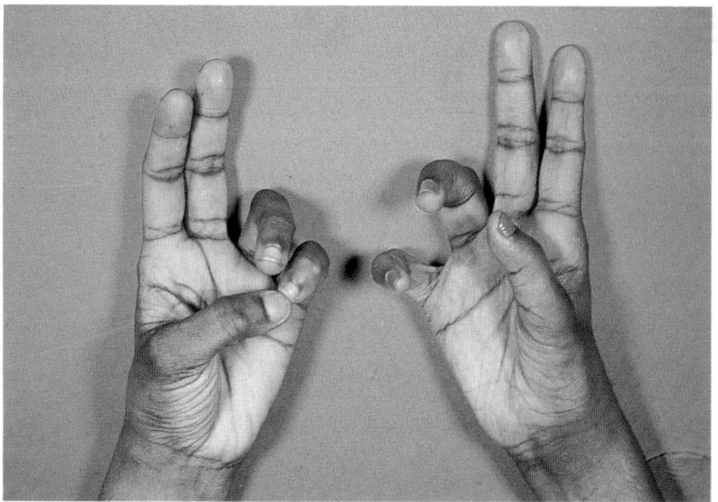

Fig. 16 Reduced power of small muscles of the right hand due to poliomyelitis.

Common cold (acute coryza)

Aetiology

Rhinoviruses mainly—there are many strains. Spread is by direct contact and droplet transmission.

Clinical features

After a 12–120 h incubation period there is a watery nasal discharge and sneezing (Fig. 17). If there is sinusitis, pyrexia and malaise may develop.

Management

Symptomatic.

Whooping cough (pertussis)

Aetiology

Bordetella pertussis.

Pathology

Spreads easily by droplets.

Clinical features

Incubation 7–10 days. Initially, there is mild pyrexia and respiratory infection and, later, cough with cyanotic spasms. Conjunctival haemorrhage can arise (Fig. 18), as can ulceration of the lingual frenulum due to persistent coughing.

Management

Special nursing during spasms.

Prevention

Vaccinate in infancy (diphtheria, pertussis, tetanus (DPT) vaccine).

Scarlet fever

Aetiology

Usually *Streptococcus pyogenes.* Droplet spread to pharynx.

Clinical features

Incubation 2–4 days followed by pharyngitis, cervical lymphadenopathy, pyrexia, headache and vomiting. A rash appears on the second day, initially on the neck, then spreading to the soles, palms and flexures and followed by desquamation.

Management

Penicillin or erythromycin.

Complications

Peritonsillar abscess, otitis media, glomerulonephritis, rheumatic fever.

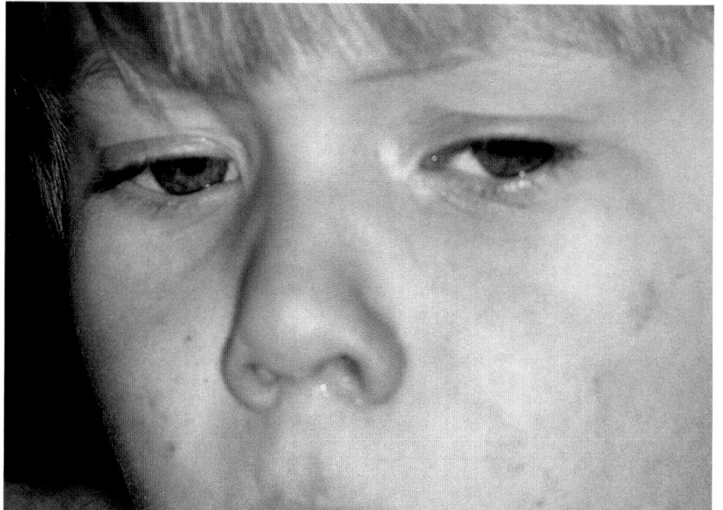

Fig. 17 Coryza.

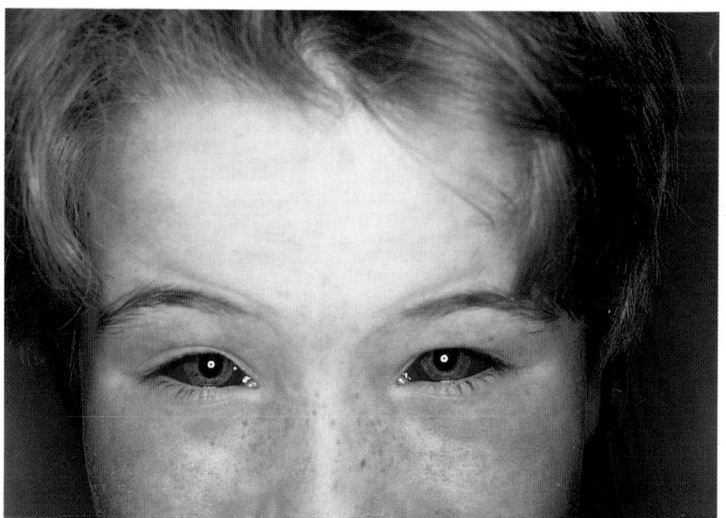

Fig. 18 Conjunctival haemorrhage in whooping cough.

Tetanus

Aetiology	*Clostridium tetani.*
Pathology	Spores found in soil and enter via a penetrating wound.
Clinical features	Incubation 5–10 days. Trismus (lockjaw), muscle stiffness and pain in the face (risus sardonicus, Fig. 19), neck or back, lead to generalized muscle spasm with arched back (opisthotonus).
Complications	Asphyxia; and autonomic instability leading to cardiac arrhythmias.
Investigations	Diagnosis *must* be clinical.
Management	Intensive care and full respiratory support. Human tetanus immunoglobulin should be given early.
Prevention	Vaccinate in infancy (DPT vaccine). Boost at 5–10 year intervals or on wounding.

Diphtheria

Aetiology	*Corynebacterium diphtheriae.*
Pathology	Dissemination is by droplets.
Clinical features	Incubation 2–4 days. Whitish pseudomembrane over tonsils can cause respiratory obstruction. Gross neck oedema (bull neck) may develop.
Complications	Myocarditis and paralyses—typically of palate, eye muscles and later diaphragm.
Investigations	Culture from throat or nose.
Management	Diphtheria antitoxin; erythromycin.
Prevention	Vaccination in infancy (DPT vaccine).

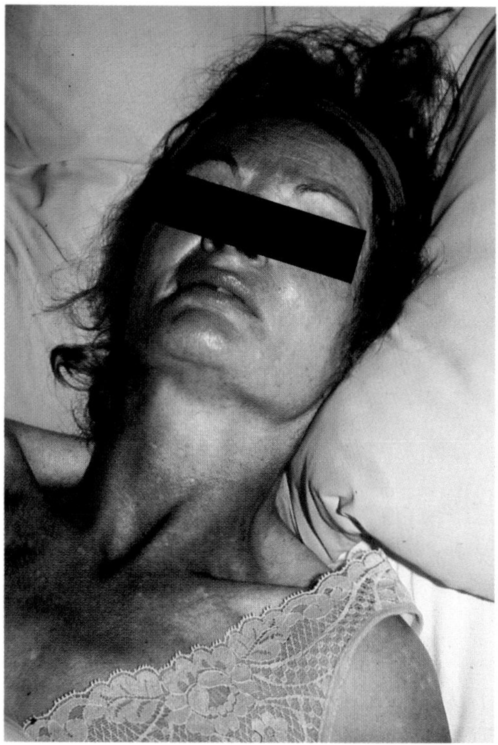

Fig. 19 Tetanus: involuntary facial muscle spasm 'risus sardonicus'.

Syphilis

Aetiology and pathology

Treponema pallidum. Syphilis is a sexually transmitted disease (STD).

Clinical features

Primary syphilis: 10–100 days' incubation; then a painless indurated ulcer (hard, Hunterian or primary chancre) develops.

Secondary syphilis: up to 12 weeks later: fever; lymphadenopathy; rash on the palms (syphilides); papules perianally (condyloma lata); and mucous patches or snail track ulcers in the mouth. Liver and CNS lesions.

Tertiary syphilis: after 2–20 years: swellings (gummas) in skin, mucosae, bone or viscera, cardiovascular disease, e.g. thoracic aortic aneurysm and neurological manifestations.

Congenital syphilis: early features include nasal snuffles and mucosal ulceration; later there is failure to thrive, dental, bony and facial anomalies and deafness (Figs 20 & 21).

Investigations

Dark ground microscopy of smear from ulcer, and serology.

Management

Procaine penicillin i.m. for 21 days. Exclude other STDs and trace contacts.

Gonorrhoea

Aetiology and pathology

Neisseria gonorrhoea: an STD. Infects columnar epithelia, e.g. urethra, cervix or rectum.

Clinical features and investigations

Incubation 2–10 days. Often asymptomatic but can include dysuria and purulent discharge (Fig. 22). Smear and culture.

Management

Penicillin or spectinomycin.

Nonspecific urethritis (non-gonococcal urethritis)

Aetiology

Chlamydia trachomatis, Mycoplasma hominis, Ureaplasma urealyticum: all common STDs.

Clinical features

Urethritis, discharge and possible later female infertility.

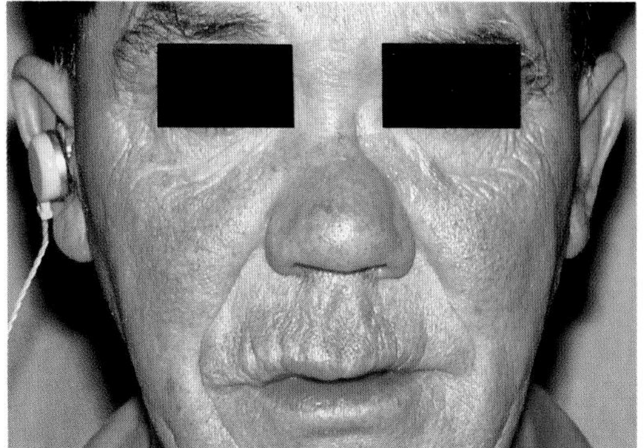

Fig. 20 Congenital syphilis: deafness, sunken nasal bridge and rhagades.

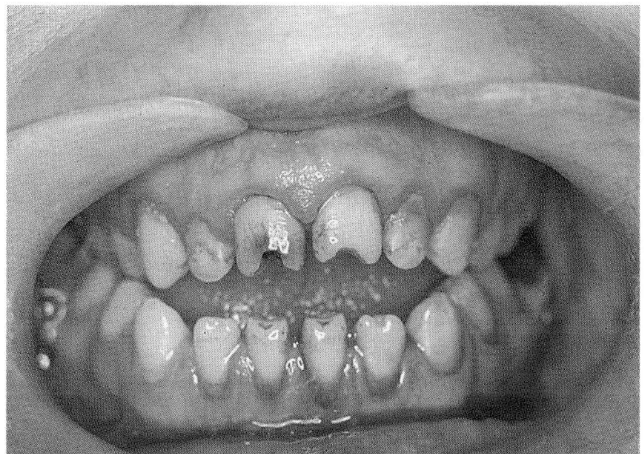

Fig. 21 Hutchinson's incisors in congenital syphilis.

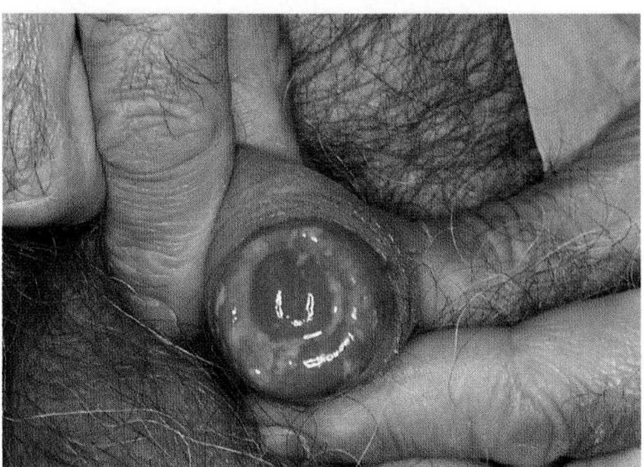

Fig. 22 Gonorrhoea: purulent urethral discharge.

Candidosis (candidiasis)

Aetiology

Candida species, usually *C. albicans*.

Pathology

Candida species are commensals that become opportunistic, particularly if local ecology changes or there is a T lymphocyte defect.

Clinical features

Oral candidosis: white papules (Fig. 23), red lesions on palate or tongue, or angular stomatitis.

Vulval/vaginal candidosis: redness, soreness or itching.

Other types: intertrigo, candidal infection of the nails (Fig. 24).

Investigations

Smear and culture.

Management

Antifungals and treat predisposing cause.

Scabies

Aetiology

The mite *Sarcoptes scabiei*. Spread by close contact.

Clinical features

Affects fingers, elbows, ankles, breasts and genitalia. The burrows form small curved tracks in the skin with a vesicle at one end (the mite). Hypersensitivity within 4–6 weeks causes itch.

Management

Gamma benzene hexachloride lotion on affected patient, partner and family members.

Lice

Aetiology

Head lice (*Pediculus humanus capitis*) (Fig. 25): usually in children, causing scalp itchiness. Body lice (*Pediculus humanus corporis*): common in socially deprived. Crabs (*Phthirus pubis*): sexually transmitted, causing perineal itchiness.

Impetigo

Aetiology

Staphylococcus aureus, *Streptococcus pyogenes* or both. They are highly contagious.

Clinical features

Vesicles which crust (Fig. 26).

Management

Systemic flucloxacillin or erythromycin.

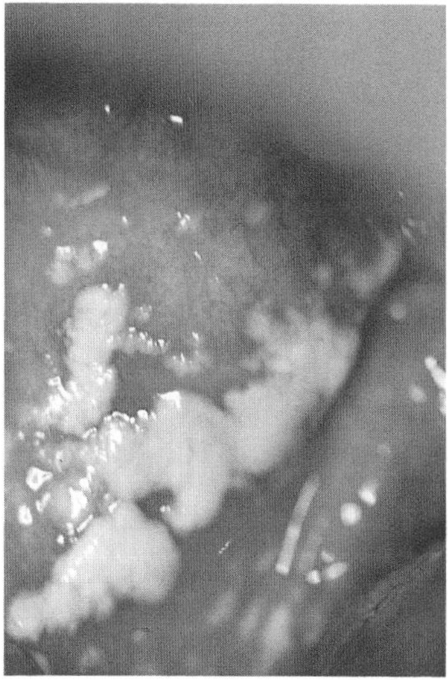

Fig. 23 Pseudomembraneous candidosis (thrush).

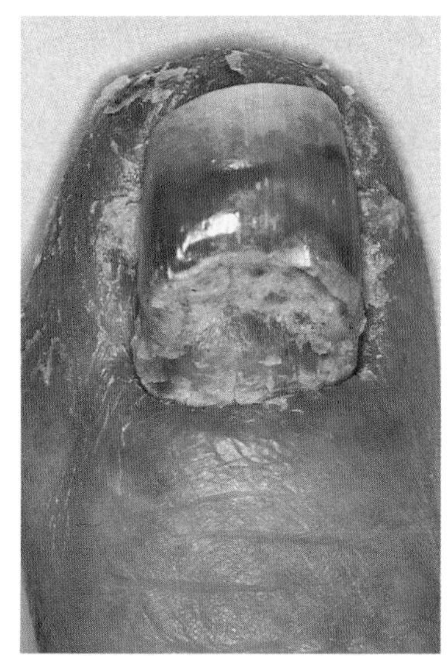

Fig. 24 Candidal infection of nails.

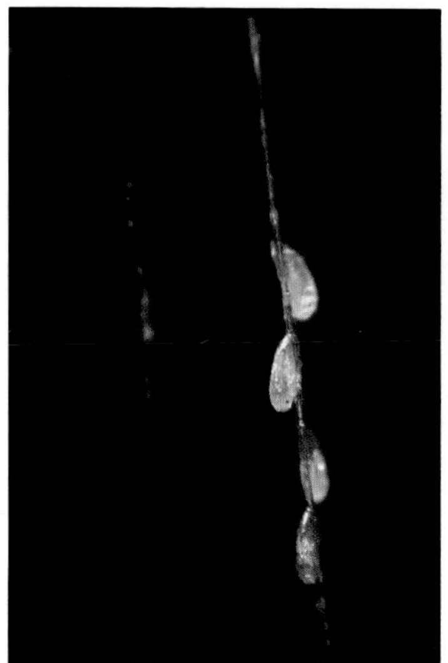

Fig. 25 Lice eggs on strand of hair.

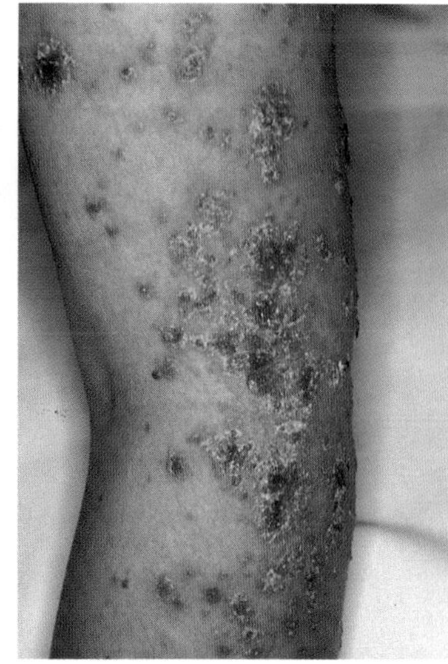

Fig. 26 Impetigo.

2 / Dermatological disease

Urticaria and angioedema

Aetiology and pathology

Mast cell release of vasoactive amines precipitated by acute hypersensitivity, chemical or physical factors.

Clinical features

Urticaria: erythematous pruritic swellings (Fig. 27).

Angioedema: swelling of lips, tongue (Fig. 28), oral mucosa, eyelids and sometimes neck, leading to airway obstruction.

Investigations

C1 esterase inhibitor assay to exclude deficiency, e.g. *hereditary* angioedema (inhibitor reduced). Skin testing may determine precipitants.

Management

- Avoid precipitants.
- H_1 antihistamine (cetirizine).
- Subcutaneous adrenaline and intravenous hydrocortisone if airway threatened.
- Emergency tracheostomy in severe angioedema.

Atopic eczema

Aetiology

Provoked by allergens in food, animal danders, house dust and pollens, and by emotional factors.

Clinical features

Infants: red papulovesicles mainly on cheeks, neck and groin.

Children: pruritic, papular and lichenified plaques mainly in antecubital and popliteal fossae (i.e. flexor surfaces). It may also present in other forms (Fig. 29).

Adults: lesions similar to those in children, but mainly at nape of neck, flexures (Fig. 30) and dorsum of hands.

Management

- Avoid allergens.
- Emollients, soap substitutes, coal tar creams.
- Topical corticosteroids (used sparingly).

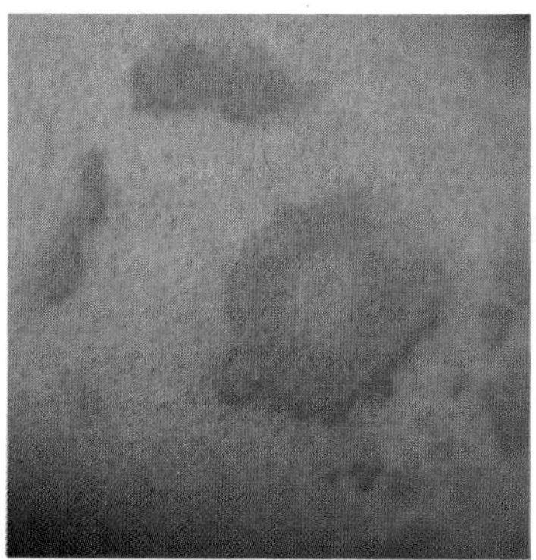

Fig. 27 Urticaria.

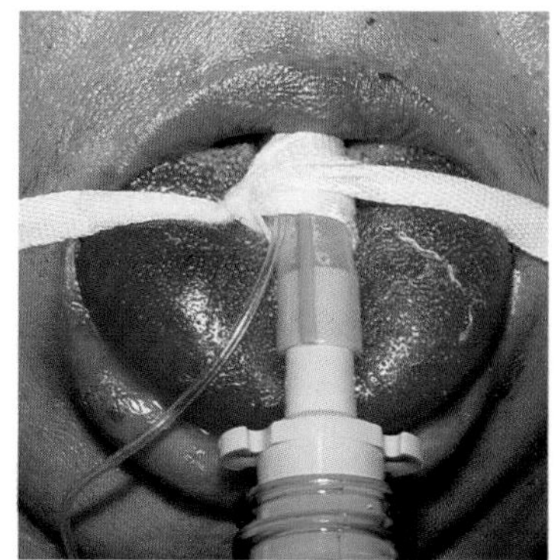

Fig. 28 Lingual swelling in angioedema.

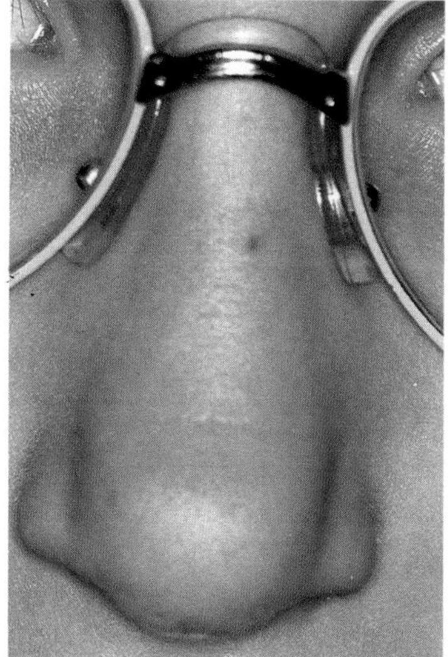

Fig. 29 Allergic salute: note the horizontal nasal skin fold in hay fever which is often seen with atopic eczema.

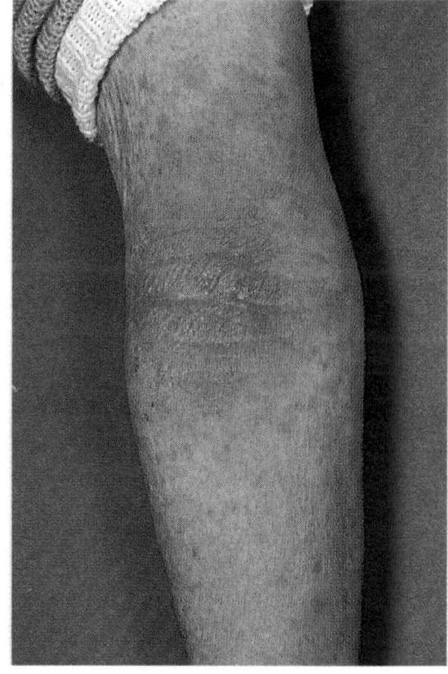

Fig. 30 Atopic eczema.

Acne vulgaris

Aetiology and pathology

Obstruction of pilosebaceous ducts, causing inflammation of sebaceous glands stimulated by androgens. *Propionibacterium acnes* and others release enzymes, aggravating inflammation.

Clinical features

Blackheads, whiteheads, pustules, papules, nodules or cysts, mainly on the face and back (Fig. 31). They may scar.

Management

Antiseptics, benzoylperoxide, keratolytics (e.g. salicyclic acid), antimicrobials, vitamin A derivatives, ultraviolet light, or dermabrasion.

Psoriasis

Aetiology

Unclear.

Clinical features

Demarcated red plaques covered by silver scales, bleeding on scratching (Auspitz's sign). Lesions occur mainly over knees and elbows (extensor surfaces, cf eczema) (Fig. 32), scalp or palms and soles. Nails are pitted (ice-pick pitting) (Fig. 33) or separated (onycholysis). Arthropathy may also be a feature.

Management

Usually topical dithranol/corticosteroids, or psoralens with UVA light (PUVA).

Lichen planus

Aetiology

Unknown. Sometimes caused by drugs or chemicals.

Pathology

T lymphocyte attack on basal stratified squamous epithelium.

Clinical features

- *Skin*—purple, pruritic, polygonal papules on flexor surfaces of wrists, and shins (Fig. 34) or sacrum.
- *Nails*—ridged.
- *Mucosae*—white, lacy, papular or erosive lesions (see Fig. 43, p. 28).

Investigations

Biopsy.

Management

Topical corticosteroids.

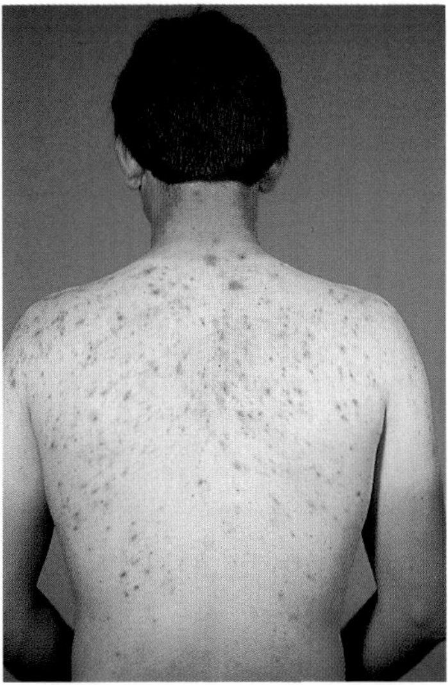

Fig. 31 Acne vulgaris of the shoulders and neck.

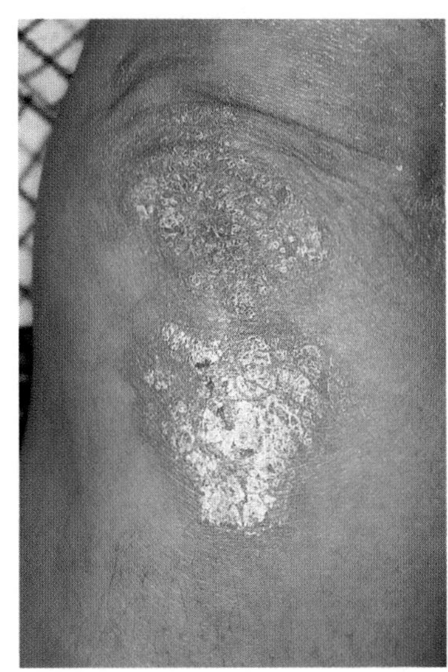

Fig. 32 Psoriasis affecting the extensor aspect of the elbow.

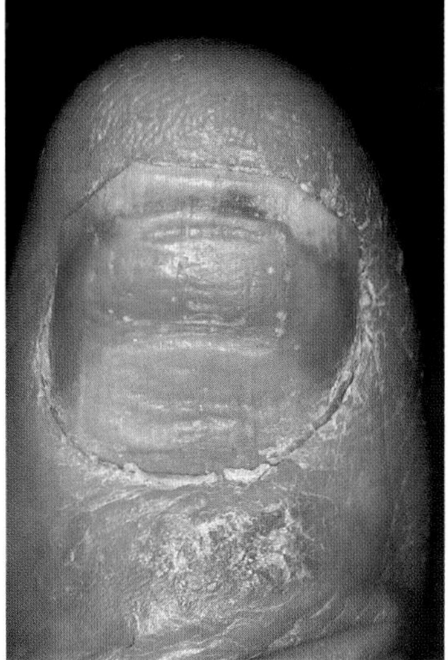

Fig. 33 Psoriasis of the nails.

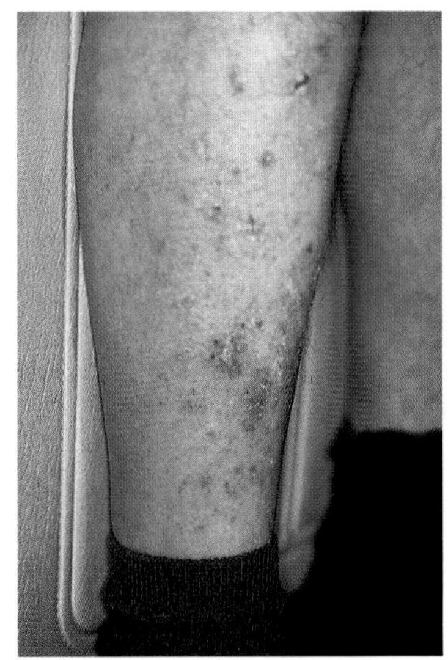

Fig. 34 Lichen planus of the extensor aspect of the lower leg.

Pemphigus

Aetiology

An autoimmune disease seen mainly in those from the Mediterranean littoral. Occasionally paraneoplastic.

Pathology

Autoantibodies against epithelial intercellular cement induce acantholysis in stratified squamous epithelium.

Clinical features

Oral ulcers and skin blisters (Fig. 35) especially where traumatized (Nikolsky's sign). There is sometimes conjunctival involvement. Pemphigus can be lethal.

Investigations/ Management

Biopsy and tests for serum autoantibodies. Exclude malignancy. Systemic immunosuppressants.

Pemphigoid

Aetiology and pathology

Autoantibodies attack basement membrane zone causing subepithelial vesiculation.

Clinical features

Mucous membrane pemphigoid: affects mouth, eye, pharynx and genitalia with blisters, ulcers and scarring.

Bullous pemphigoid: skin blisters.

Investigations/ Management

Similar to pemphigus. Topical or systemic corticosteroids.

Erythema multiforme

Aetiology

Usually unclear but may be triggered by herpes simplex, mycoplasma, sulphonamides, cephalosporins or barbiturates.

Pathology

Serum immune complexes with sub- and/or intra-epithelial vesiculation.

Clinical features

- *Skin*—target (iris) lesions.
- *Mucosae*—conjunctivitis; swollen blood-stained lips (Fig. 36) and oral ulceration; genital ulceration.

Management

Systemic corticosteroids or aciclovir.

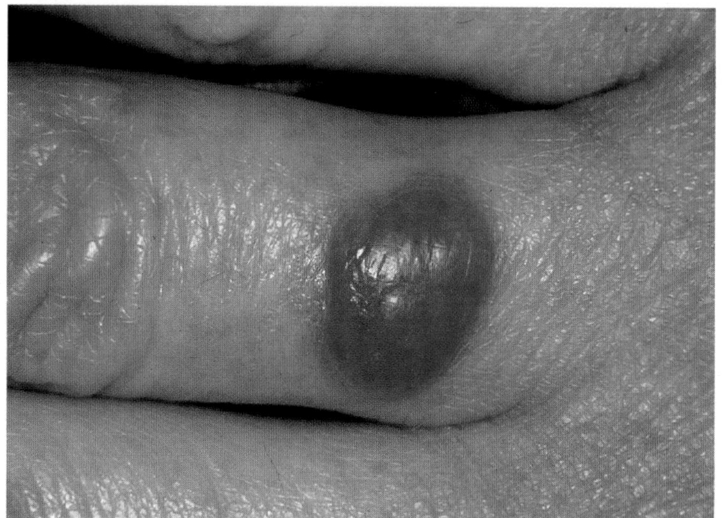

Fig. 35 Pemphigus vulgaris.

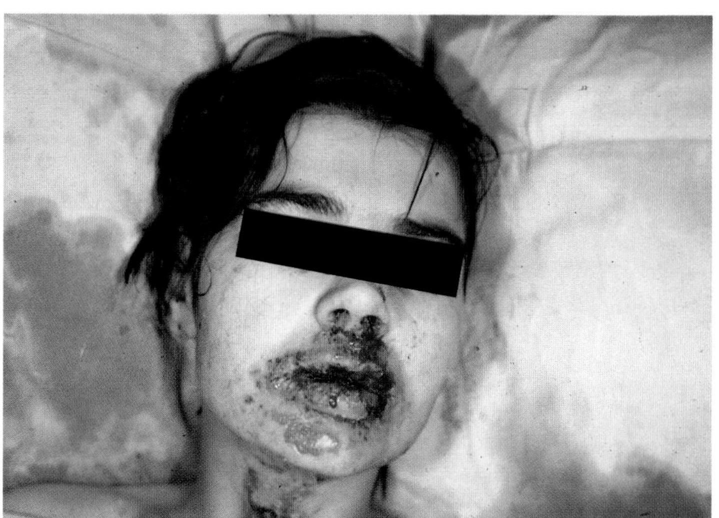

Fig. 36 Erythema multiforme causing blood-encrusted lips.

Basal cell carcinoma

Aetiology and pathology — Possibly due to sun exposure; locally aggressive but no metastases.

Clinical features — Involves mid-face and periorbital sites mainly. Appears as a papule with pearly surface and telangiectasia (Fig. 37); later there is ulceration and crusting.

Investigations — Biopsy.

Management — Excision or radiotherapy.

Squamous cell carcinoma

Aetiology and pathology — Long-term sun exposure; can metastasize.

Clinical features — Hyperkeratotic, crusted area (Fig. 38); may ulcerate with typical rolled edge, or fungate (Fig. 39).

Investigations — Biopsy.

Management — Surgical excision with or without radiotherapy.

Malignant melanoma

Aetiology and pathology — Intense episodes of sun exposure. Lesions can arise de novo or from pre-existing naevi. Spread is rapid producing satellite deposits, lymph node and other metastases.

Clinical features — Increase in size, or change in outline, colour, or consistency of pigmented areas (Fig. 40). Ulceration, pruritus and bleeding are strongly suspicious.

Investigations — Wide excisional biopsy.

Management — Chemotherapy may be of additional benefit in widespread disease.

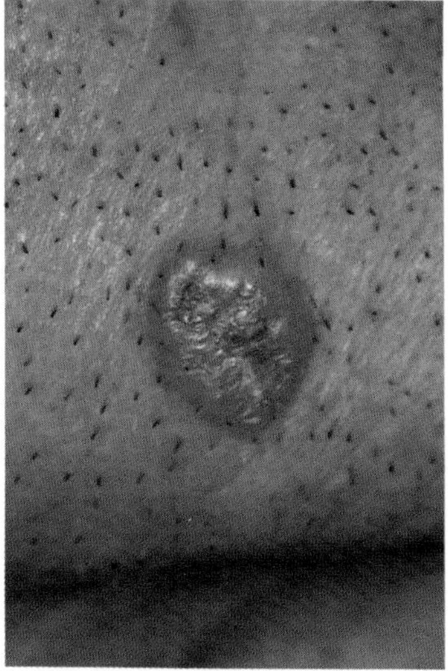

Fig. 37 Basal cell carcinoma.

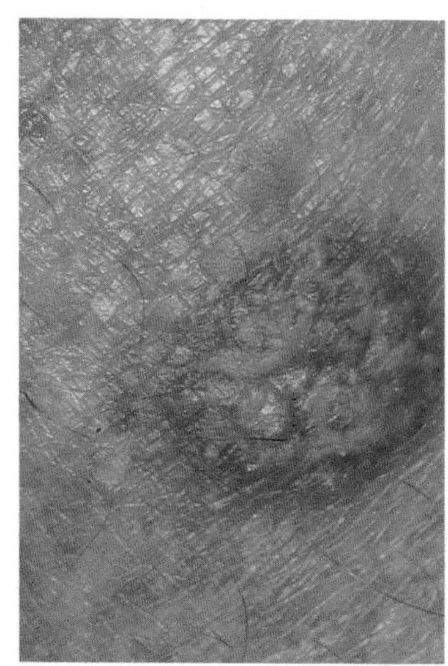

Fig. 38 Small squamous cell carcinoma.

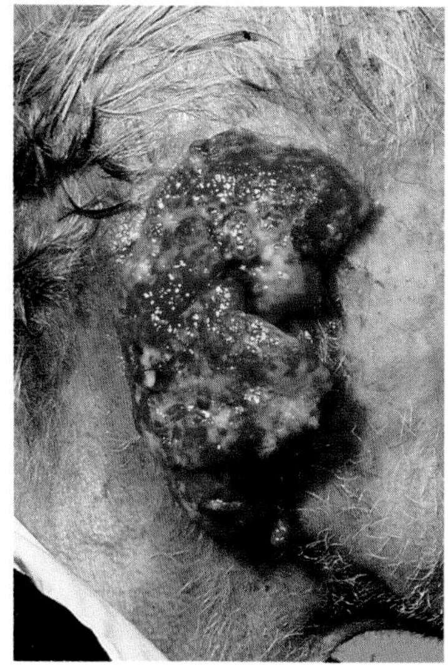

Fig. 39 Large fungating squamous cell carcinoma of the auricle.

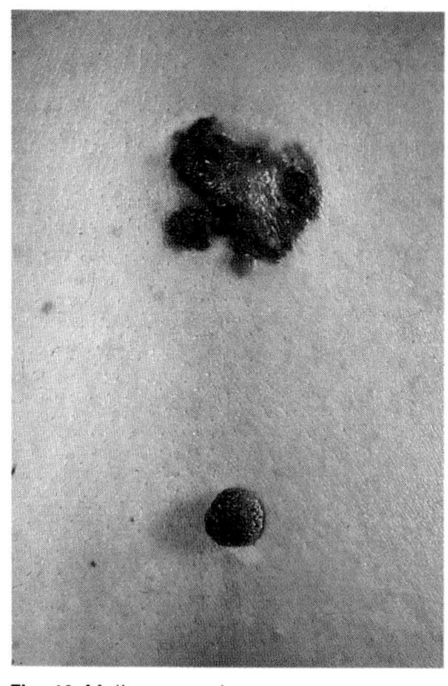

Fig. 40 Malignant melanoma.

3 / Cardiovascular disease

Hypertension

Definition

Persistent elevation of systemic blood pressure—usually diastolic greater than 95 mmHg, systolic greater than 160 mmHg.

Epidemiology

Common; develops mainly in middle to late life.

Aetiology

In 95% there is no identifiable aetiological factor (i.e. essential hypertension). Obesity, arteriosclerosis and high salt intake aggravate the disorder. Secondary hypertension occurs in endocrine (e.g. hyperaldosteronism) or renal disease.

Clinical features

Pronounced apex beat (left ventricular hypertrophy), loud second heart sound (aortic valve snaps shut). Retinal vascular changes result in haemorrhage and swelling of the optic disc (papilloedema).

Investigations

- Blood pressure (BP) measurements (Fig. 41).
- Electrocardiogram (ECG)—left ventricular hypertrophy (Fig. 42).
- Urea and electrolytes—renal/endocrine causes.
- Blood lipids—underlying arteriosclerotic tendency.

Management

- Weight loss.
- Regular exercise.
- Reduced salt, alcohol and smoking.
- Diuretics, β-blockers (can cause oral lichen planus (Fig. 43)), angiotensin converting enzyme inhibitors or calcium antagonists (may cause gingival hyperplasia).
- Strive for a steady blood pressure of <150/95 (systolic/diastolic).

Prognosis

Effective treatment improves prognosis. *Malignant hypertension* is a rapidly rising, or very high, blood pressure. If not corrected, death within 1 year is likely.

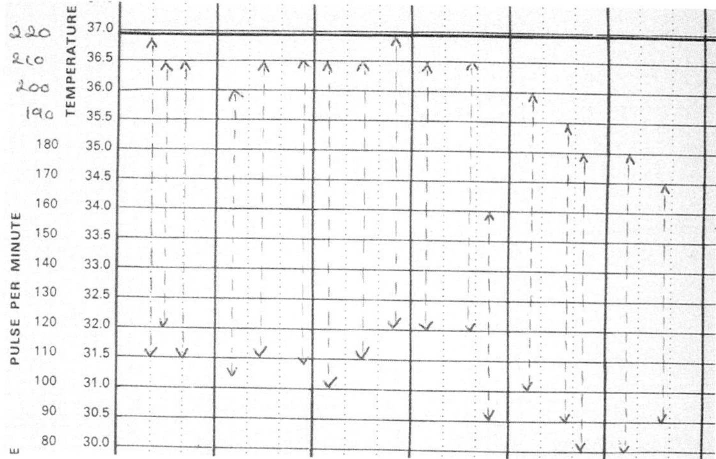

Fig. 41 Hypertension: only diagnosed by repeated measurement of blood pressure.

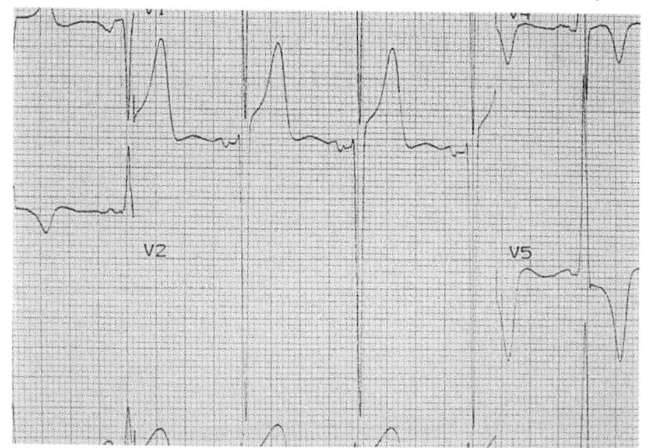

Fig. 42 ECG changes indicating left ventricular hypertrophy.

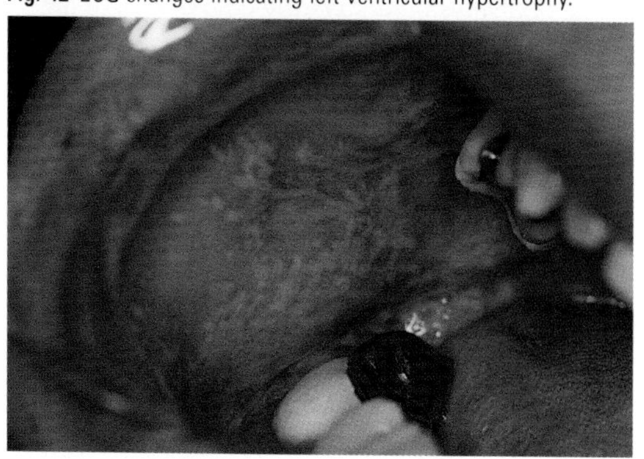

Fig. 43 Oral lichen planus caused by β-blockers.

Congenital heart disease

Aetiology

Usually of unknown cause but maternal alcohol or drug abuse, drug therapy, radiation, infection (e.g. rubella) and chromosomal anomalies (Down syndrome) may be responsible.

Classification

Classified as acyanotic or cyanotic (Fig. 44, Table 1).

Clinical features

Poor feeding, failure to thrive, clubbing, squatting, syncope and cardiac failure.

Management

Similar to cardiac failure (p. 37), plus cardiac surgery.

Atherosclerosis (arteriosclerosis)

Aetiology

Smoking, diabetes mellitus, obesity and hyperlipidaemia (Fig. 45) predispose. A familial pattern may reflect social or dietary habits or an hyperlipidaemia.

Pathology

- Atheromatous plaques with secondary thrombotic occlusion.
- Aneurysm formation, commonly at coronary arteries, carotid bifurcation, aorto-iliac region (Fig. 46, p. 32), superficial femoral or popliteal artery.

Clinical features

Calf pain on exercise (claudication). Aneurysm of the abdominal aorta can be an incidental finding or can rupture. Carotid involvement may cause transient ischaemic attacks (TIAs) or cerebrovascular accidents (CVAs). Sudden arterial occlusion can give rise to a painful, paraesthetic, pulseless, persistently cold and pale limb (5 'p's).

Investigations

- Ultrasound, plain radiography and computerized axial tomography (CT) for aorta.
- Doppler studies and arteriography for other vessels.

Management

Modify lifestyle; lipid lowering agents. Angioplasty to remove plaques and/or open up vessels. Graft bypass of obliterated vessels.

Table 1 **Common congenital cardiac disorders**

Acyanotic	Cyanotic
Ventricular septal defects (various) Atrial septal defects (usually ostium secundum) Patent ductus arteriosus—persistent blood flow from aorta into pulmonary artery Coarctation of aorta—constriction of aorta near level of ligamentum arteriosum (distal to left subclavian artery)	Fallot's tetralogy, i.e. • right ventricular enlargement • restricted right ventricular outflow • ventricular septal defect (VSD) • aorta positioned over VSD Transposition of major vessels—pulmonary arteries arise from left ventricle, and aorta from right ventricle

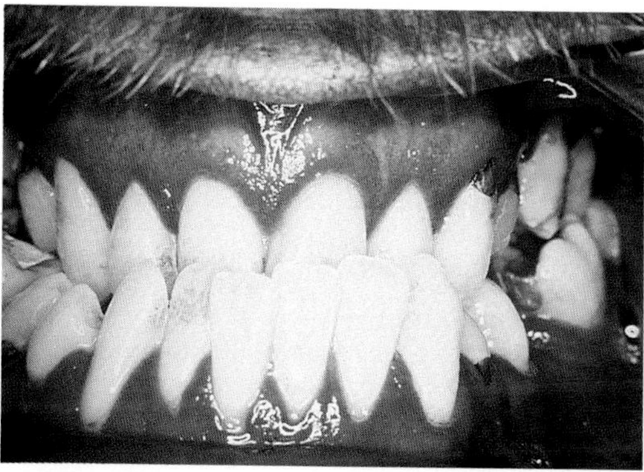

Fig. 44 Gingival cyanosis in right to left cardioc shunt.

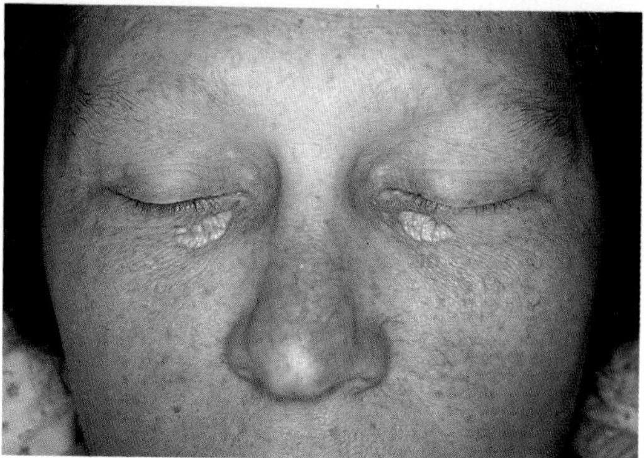

Fig. 45 Xanthelasma: lipid deposits in skin caused by hyperlipidaemia.

Ischaemic heart disease

Aetiology

Coronary atherosclerosis (arteriosclerosis).

Clinical features

Angina pectoris: chest pain radiating to neck or left arm precipitated by exercise, emotion or cold. Relieved by rest or vasodilators.

Myocardial infarction (MI): pain, like angina, but more severe or persistent (e.g. more than 30 min), may be accompanied by nausea, vomiting, sweating and possibly loss of consciousness. The pain is unrelieved by vasodilators. *Sudden death* may ensue.

Investigations

- ECG (Fig. 47).
- Cardiac enzymes—raised in infarction.
- Chest radiograph—pulmonary oedema.

Management

Angina:
- avoid precipitants
- glyceryl trinitrate (sublingual) for pain
- prophylactic β-blockers and nitrates
- angioplasty for atheromas in proximal coronary vessels
- bypass surgery for multivessel disease.

Myocardial infarction:
- aspirin and oxygen and antiemetics
- analgesia (e.g. morphine)
- thrombolysis (e.g. streptokinase)
- 24 h bed rest
- avoid constipation
- correct arrhythmias or failure
- later, investigate extent of infarct
- later, consider suitability for surgery.

Complications

Angina may go on to MI. Complications of MI include: cardiac arrhythmias and failure; thrombi and emboli; rupture of valvular chordae; serositis.

Prognosis

Over 30% of MI victims die within 2 h. 90% of remainder are alive at 1 year and by 10 years 40% are alive.

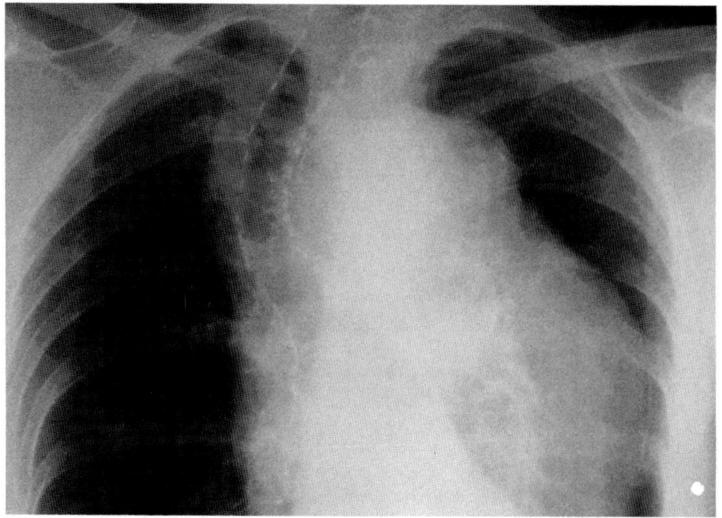

Fig. 46 Arteriosclerotic aortic aneurysm with displacement of the trachea.

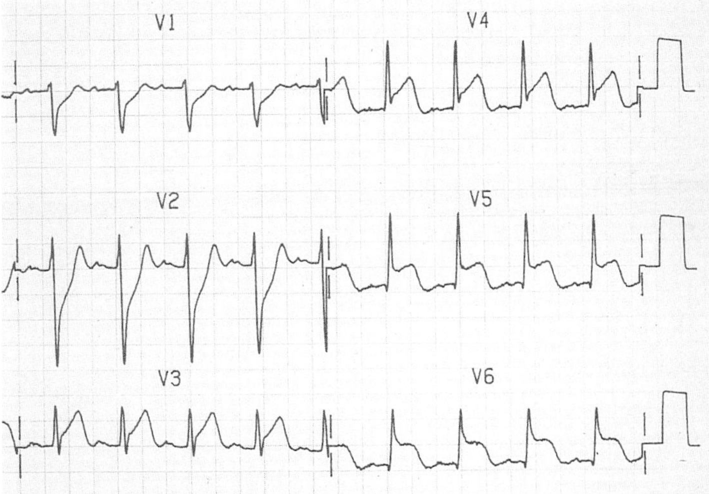

Fig. 47 ST elevation in ECG from myocardial infarction.

Rheumatic fever

Definition

Inflammatory disease of the layers of the heart (i.e. endocardium, myocardium and pericardium). Rheumatic fever also affects skin, joints and central nervous system.

Epidemiology

Usually occurs in 5–15-year-olds. It is declining in the West but still common in the Middle East, Far East, South America and Eastern Europe.

Aetiology

Initial pharyngeal *Streptococcus pyogenes A* infection gives rise to production of antibodies that cross-react with cardiac, joint, skin and CNS tissues.

Clinical features

- Flitting polyarthritis of the large joints.
- Carditis (e.g. pain, acute failure, murmurs).
- Choreiform movements (Sydenham's chorea; St Vitus' dance).
- Erythema marginatum—transient pink rash (Fig. 48).
- Subcutaneous nodules—pea-sized, over tendons, joints and bony prominences.
- Other features include fever, arthralgia, raised erythrocyte sedimentation rate (ESR) and C reactive protein (CRP), leucocytosis, cardiac conduction anomalies, and associated features (Fig. 49).

Management

- Bed rest.
- Penicillin G in acute stage, thereafter penicillin V orally as prophylaxis until 20 years of age or 5 years after last attack.
- High dose salicylates.
- Corticosteroids (occasionally for carditis).

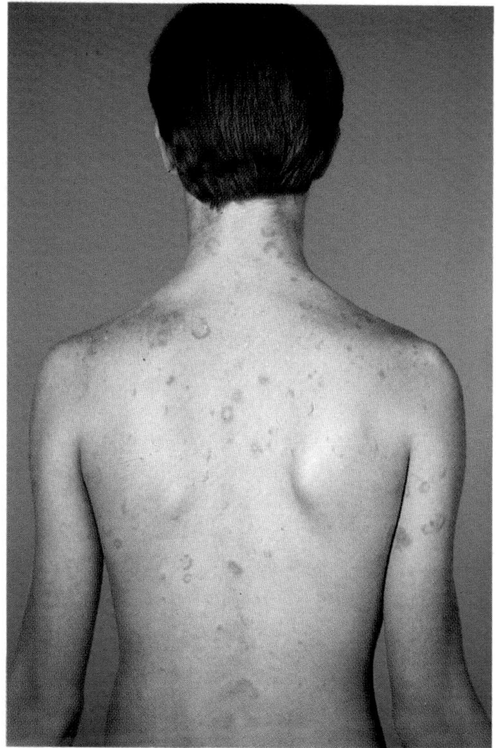

Fig. 48 Erythema marginatum in acute rheumatic fever.

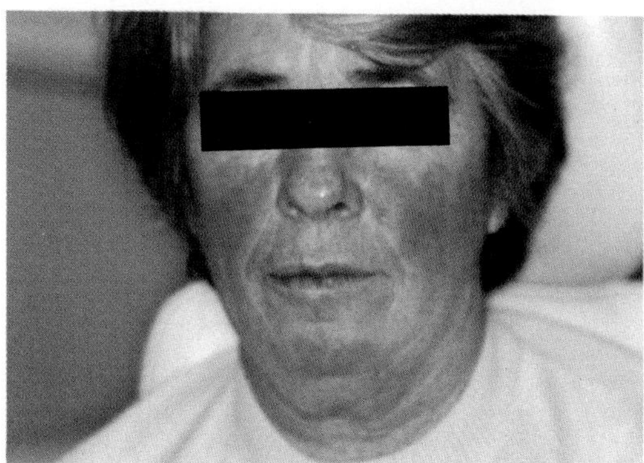

Fig. 49 Malar flush can be a feature of mitral stenosis secondary to chronic rheumatic carditis.

Infective endocarditis

Definition

Infection of the endocardium.

Aetiology

Common causative organisms include *Streptococcus viridans, Staphylococcus aureus, Streptococcus faecalis* and other streptococci. Dental procedures are the source of 10% of cases (usually *Strep. viridans*). In 5% no causative agent is found. The infecting microbes in blood settle on damaged valve leaflets, forming vegetations. Embolization of infective material or immune complexes cause other features.

Clinical features

Can manifest as an acute infection or a subacute disorder subsequent to a suppurative illness. Typically there is fever, new or changing cardiac murmurs and the results of embolization and:

- anaemia, fatigue, weakness, arthromyalgia
- clubbing (Fig. 50)
- cardiac failure or murmurs
- mucosal petechiae—in conjunctivae, pharynx, retinae (Roth's spots)
- erythematous patches (Janeway lesions) on palms
- splinter haemorrhages beneath nails (Figs 51 & 52) and purpura
- Osler's nodes (hard, red, tender lesions on fingers)
- splenomegaly
- cerebral abscesses and cerebrovascular accidents
- renal lesions—causing haematuria
- arthralgia of major joints.

Management

Echocardiogram, blood cultures. Antibiotics. Occasionally valvular surgery is required. Always consider antibiotic prophylaxis for invasive dental procedures for at-risk patients.

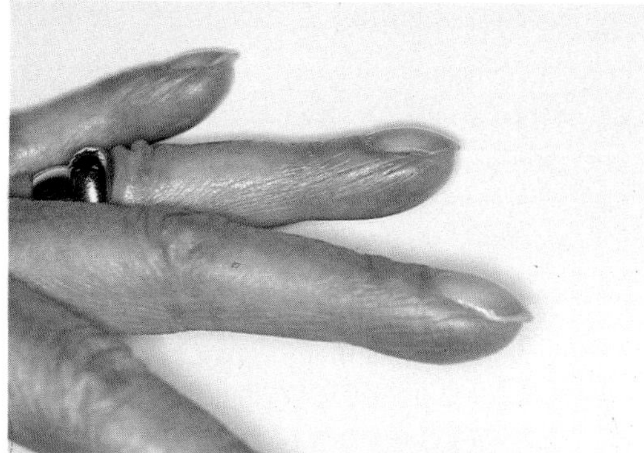

Fig. 50 Clubbing: a late effect of endocarditis.

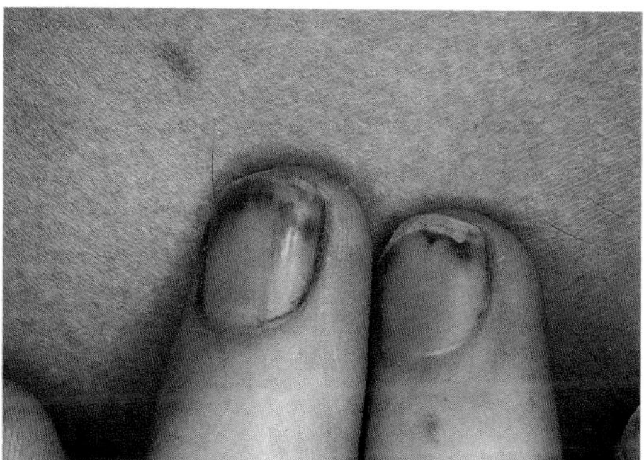

Fig. 51 Gross splinter haemorrhages in acute infective endocarditis.

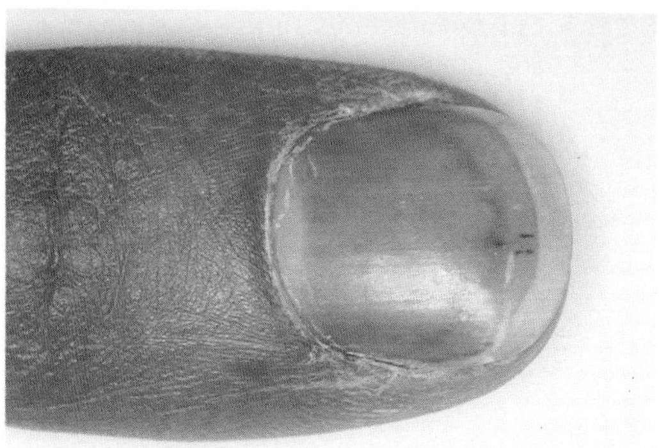

Fig. 52 Mild splinter haemorrhages are usually caused by trauma in otherwise healthy people.

Cardiac failure

Definition Insufficient cardiac output but normal venous return.

Aetiology Table 2.

Clinical features *Right-sided failure:* distended jugular veins (Fig. 53), enlarged tender liver, ascites, pitting oedema (Fig. 54), anorexia and 'gallop' cardiac rhythm.

Left-sided failure: fatigue, weakness, dyspnoea, 'gallop' cardiac rhythm, paroxysmal nocturnal dyspnoea, pulmonary oedema.

Congestive cardiac failure: right-sided failure subsequent to left-sided failure.

Management Weight reduction, low salt diet, diuretics, vasodilators, digoxin if in atrial fibrillation.

Varicose veins

Definition Pathologically dilated and tortuous veins (usually saphenous).

Aetiology Primary valve defect within the perforating veins. Prolonged standing, and raised intra-abdominal pressure—due to obesity, multiparity or pelvic and abdominal neoplasia—predispose.

Clinical features

- Dilated, tortuous, elongated, superficial leg veins.
- Eczema of the lower calf and/or chronic ulceration (Fig. 55 & Fig. 56, p. 40).

Investigations Doppler ultrasound.

Management

- *Conservative measures*—elastic support stockings, avoidance of prolonged standing.
- *Surgery*—sclerotherapy; or ligation or multiple avulsion of affected vein.

Table 2 Causes of cardiac failure

Myocardial disease	**Mechanical defects**
Ischaemic heart disease (e.g. MI)	Ventricular aneurysm
Cardiomyopathy	**Cardiac arrhythmias**
Valvular disease	Atrial fibrillation
Valvular regurgitation	Some tachycardias
Obstructed outflow	**High output failure**
Aortic stenosis	Paget's disease
Hypertension	Anaemia
Pulmonary hypertension*	Thyrotoxicosis
Restricted cardiac filling	Left to right shunt
Restrictive cardiomyopathy	
Constrictive pericarditis	
Pericardial tamponade	

**Can lead to cor pulmonale (right-sided failure subsequent to chronic pulmonary hypertension)*

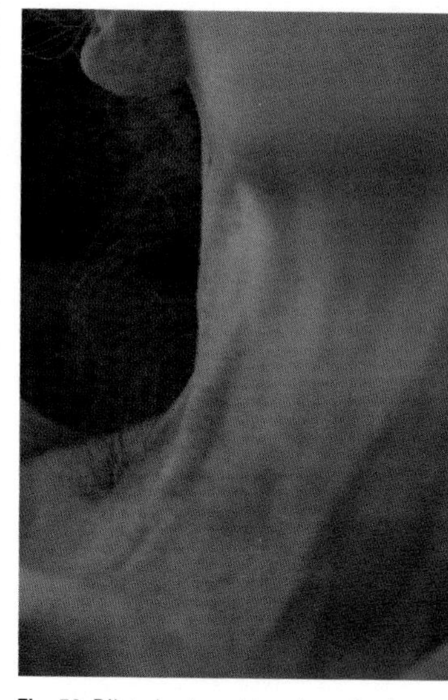

Fig. 53 Dilated external jugular veins in right-sided cardiac failure.

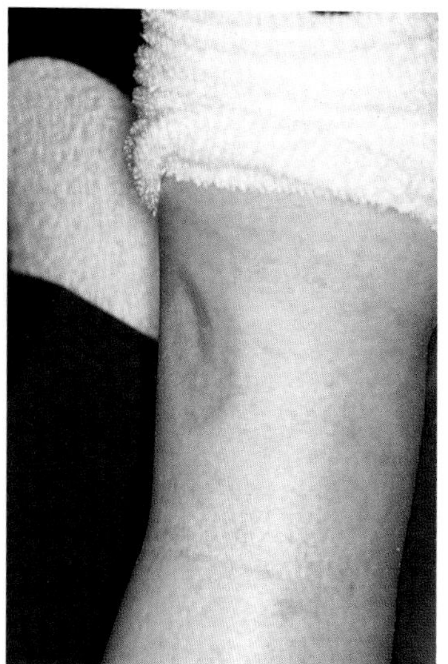

Fig. 54 Severe pitting oedema.

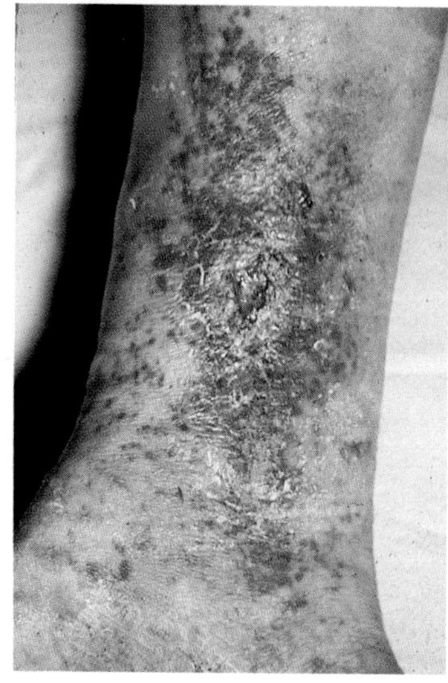

Fig. 55 Haemosiderin deposition, eczematoid change and varicose ulceration.

Deep vein thrombosis (DVT)

Aetiology

Often arises spontaneously but longstanding immobility, old age, malignancy and the oestrogen contraceptive pill predispose.

Clinical features

- Can be symptomless, or may present with secondary effects (Fig. 57) or with pulmonary embolism.
- Calf swelling and pain which is worse on dorsiflexion of foot (Homans' sign).

Investigations

Venography and Doppler analysis.

Management

Anticoagulation, mobilization and placement of a pressure elastic stocking; investigate cause.

Pulmonary embolus

Aetiology

Deep vein thrombosis, mural thrombus or atrial fibrillation. Predisposed by pelvic surgery and pregnancy.

Pathology

Embolus blocks the pulmonary artery leading to collapse, and hypoxaemia. Sometimes fatal (Fig. 58). Small emboli may cause infarction in peripheral lung sites.

Clinical features

- Dyspnoea (small embolus) or circulatory collapse (large embolism).
- Pleuritic chest pain with or without dyspnoea.

Investigations

- Chest radiograph.
- White blood cells (leukocytosis); ESR raised; blood gases (hypoxaemia and hypercapnia).
- ECG and ventilation–perfusion (V/Q) scanning.

Management

Anticoagulation and thrombolytic agents; embolectomy rarely.

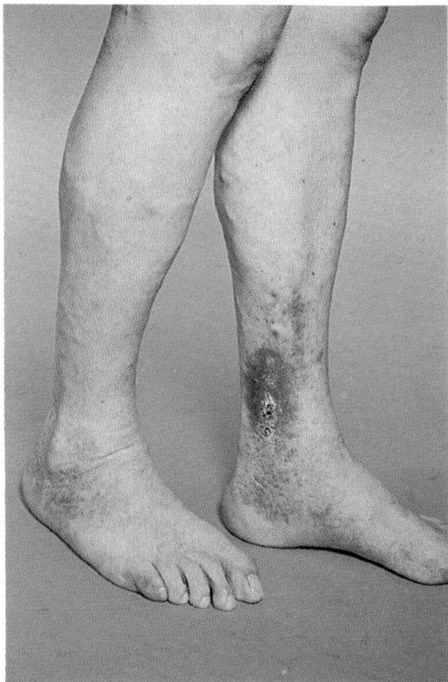

Fig. 56 Typical varicose changes on inner aspects of the lower leg.

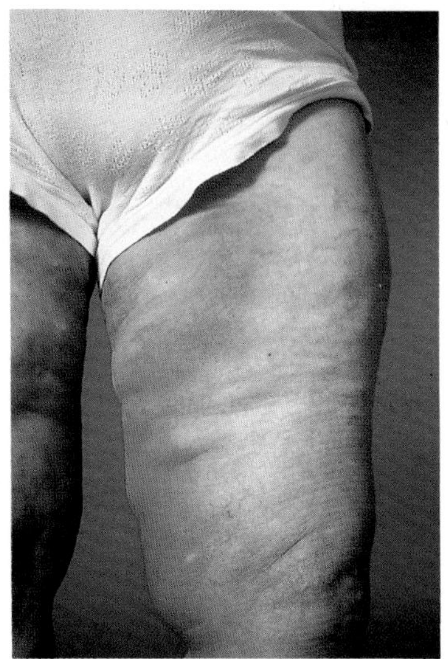

Fig. 57 Thrombophlebitis of the inner aspect of the thigh secondary to DVT.

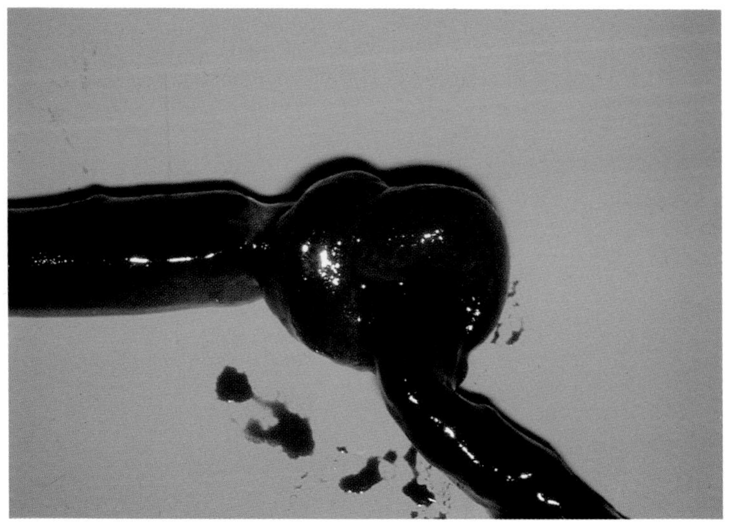

Fig. 58 Postmortem pulmonary embolus specimen.

4 / Respiratory disease

Chronic bronchitis and emphysema

Definitions

Chronic bronchitis: a *clinical* diagnosis—productive cough on most days for at least 3 months for more than 1 year.

Emphysema: a *pathological* diagnosis—dilatation and destruction of alveolar sacs with loss of surface area for gas exchange (Fig. 59).

Chronic bronchitis and emphysema usually co-exist.

Aetiology

Smoking is the main aetiological factor (Figs 60 & 61).

Clinical features

- Chronic productive cough, wheeze and dyspnoea.
- Pursing of lips during expiration.
- Exaggerated use of accessory respiratory muscles.
- Possible central cyanosis due to anoxia.

Investigations

- Lung function—limited airflow.
- Chest radiograph—overinflation of lungs.
- Blood—secondary polycythaemia, hypoxia, hypercapnia and reduced blood pH in late disease.
- ECG—right ventricular hypertrophy.

Management

Stop smoking. Bronchodilators, corticosteroids (occasionally), antibiotics and mucolytics are used in treatment. Oxygen therapy may slow progression.

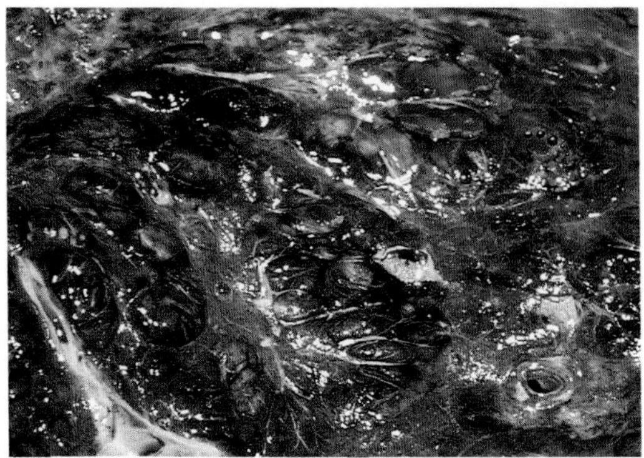

Fig. 59 Postmortem specimen showing emphysematous changes.

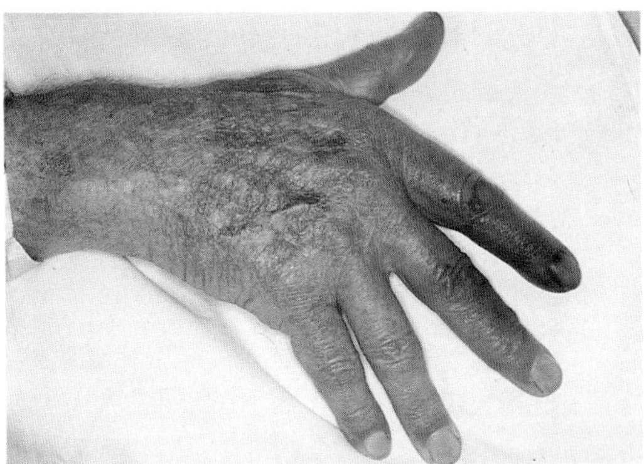

Fig. 60 Tar stains of the fingers (nicotine is colourless and does *not* stain).

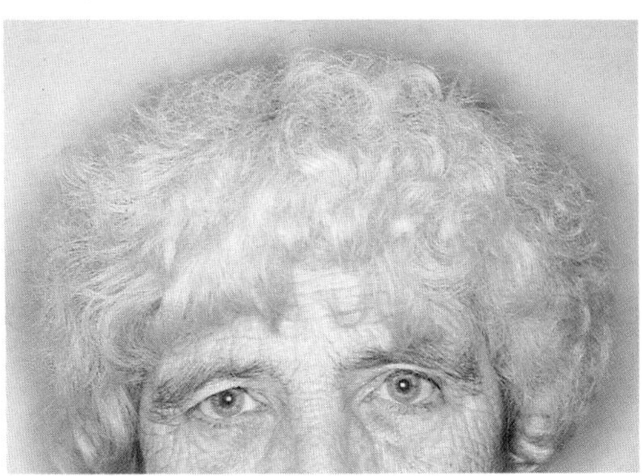

Fig. 61 Discoloration of the hair caused by smoking.

Bronchiectasis

Definition

Abnormal dilatation and thickening of bronchiolar walls, with defective mucociliary transport.

Aetiology

Usually secondary to cystic fibrosis, heavy smoking or recurrent severe respiratory tract infections.

Clinical features

Intermittent fever and productive cough (Fig. 62); persistent halitosis; failure to thrive; haemoptysis; clubbing (Fig. 63) and dyspnoea.

Investigations

Chest radiographs with or without bronchograms.

Management

- Postural drainage and physiotherapy.
- Antibiotics, bronchodilators.
- Surgery—only for localized lesions.

Cystic fibrosis (fibrocystic disease)

Definition

Autosomal recessive gene (usually) giving rise to defective cell membrane transport.

Pathology

Excessive, abnormal mucus in the respiratory and gastrointestinal tracts, causing respiratory and pancreatic insufficiency.

Clinical features

Meconium ileus in newborn; failure to thrive (Fig. 64); malabsorption and bronchiectasis. Male infertility results from obstruction of the vas deferens and epididymis; there is amenorrhoea in females.

Investigations

Elevated sodium in sweat and saliva; elevated faecal fats.

Management

- Pancreatic enzyme and vitamin supplements.
- Prophylactic antibiotics.
- Genetic counselling.

Prognosis

Improving but most patients succumb to severe respiratory infection after the 3rd decade.

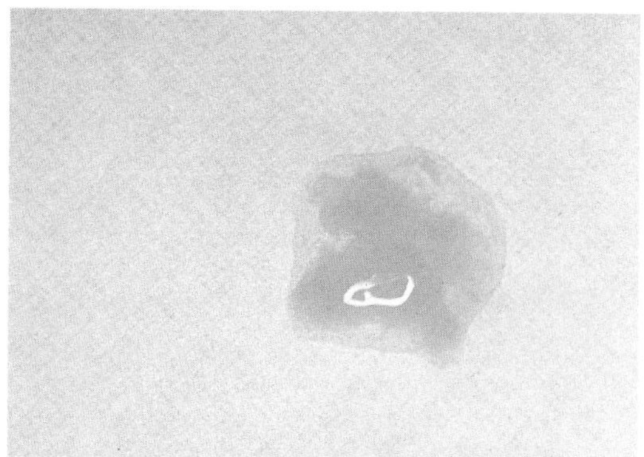

Fig. 62 Purulent sputum in bronchiectasis.

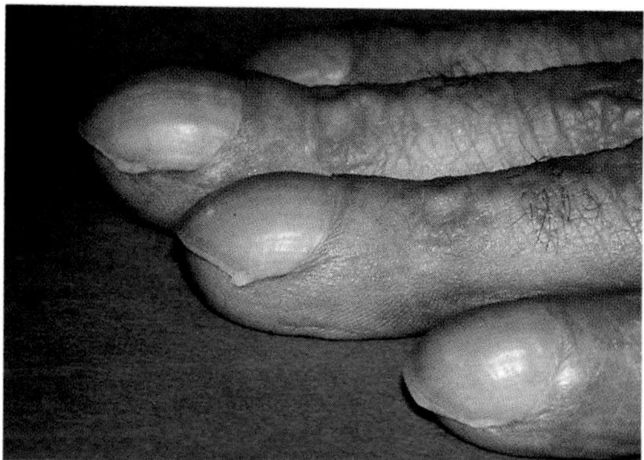

Fig. 63 Gross clubbing.

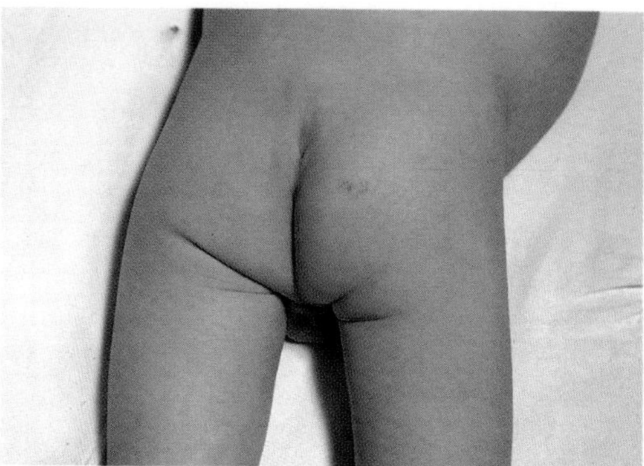

Fig. 64 Muscle wasting in cystic fibrosis.

Asthma

Definition

Intermittent, partial obstruction of the bronchi and bronchioles.

Aetiology

Airway hyper-reactivity to non-specific agents (*intrinsic* asthma) in most. Others have hypersensitivity reactions to known allergens (*extrinsic* asthma) and often a family history of other atopic disorders.

Precipitating factors

Include: exercise; cold air; emotion; drugs; allergens (e.g. pollen, house mite faeces, fungal spores, proteolytic enzymes, occupational agents, air pollution).

Clinical features

Intermittent wheeze, dyspnoea and cough.

Investigations

- Lung function—restricted airflow (Fig. 65).
- Eosinophilia and raised eosinophil count in sputum.
- Raised serum IgE.

Management

- Avoidance of stimuli—hyposensitization is rarely of any value.
- Drugs—a combination of bronchodilators (β_2-agonists—salbutamol), anticholinergics (ipratropium bromide), xanthines (theophylline or aminophylline), mast cell stabilizers (sodium cromoglycate), antihistamines (ketotifen) and corticosteroids (Fig. 66).

Complications

Status asthmaticus, i.e. tachycardia, pulsus paradoxicus and absent wheeze (due to poor airflow).

Prognosis

Extrinsic asthma tends to improve with age but asthma of late onset can be highly resistant to therapy.

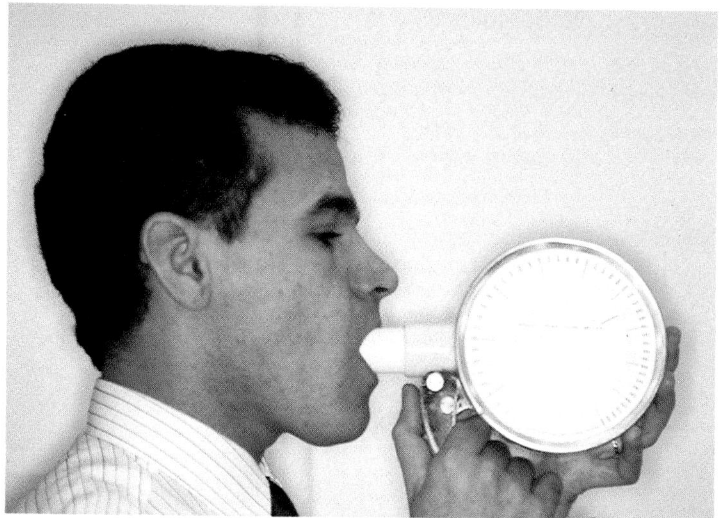

Fig. 65 Peak expiratory flows are regularly measured in asthma.

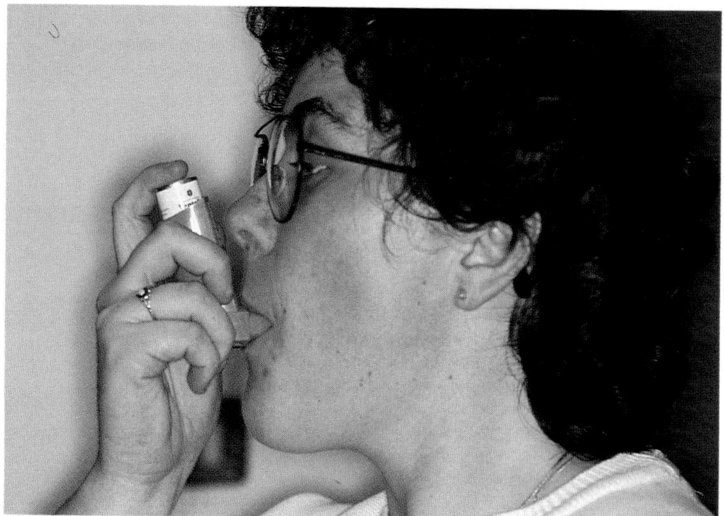

Fig. 66 β-adrenergic and corticosteroid inhalers are commonly used in the management of asthma.

Sarcoidosis

Definition and epidemiology

Multisystem granulomatous disease; more common in cities and in South East USA.

Clinical features

Acute sarcoidosis: bilateral hilar lymphadenopathy and erythema nodosum (HAEN).

Chronic sarcoidosis: (Table 3, Fig. 67).

Investigations

- Transbronchial or lesional biopsy—non-caseating granulomas.
- Blood—raised serum angiotensin converting enzyme (SACE), lysozyme and calcium.
- Chest radiography—hilar node enlargement and, in chronic disease, diffuse lung fibrosis (Fig. 68).
- Lung function—restricted.
- Loss of Mantoux reaction.

Management

No treatment in mild, asymptomatic disease. Others are treated with systemic corticosteroids and/or immunosuppressives.

Pneumonia

Definition

Inflammation of lung parenchyma.

Aetiology

Infection (Table 4), but chemicals, radiation or allergies may be causes. The disease is more common with old age, immune defect, smoking, alcohol, bronchiectasis, bronchial obstruction.

Clinical features

Fever, malaise, dyspnoea, tachypnoea, pleuritic pain, limited chest movements over affected area, increased dullness on percussion, bronchial breath sounds, increased vocal resonance, fine crackles on auscultation.

Investigations

- Chest radiographs—areas of radio-opacity (Fig. 69, Fig. 70, p. 50).
- Blood—leukocytosis, raised ESR, bacterial culture.
- Sputum culture and sensitivity.

Management

Antimicrobials.

Complications

Lung collapse, abscess; pneumothorax.

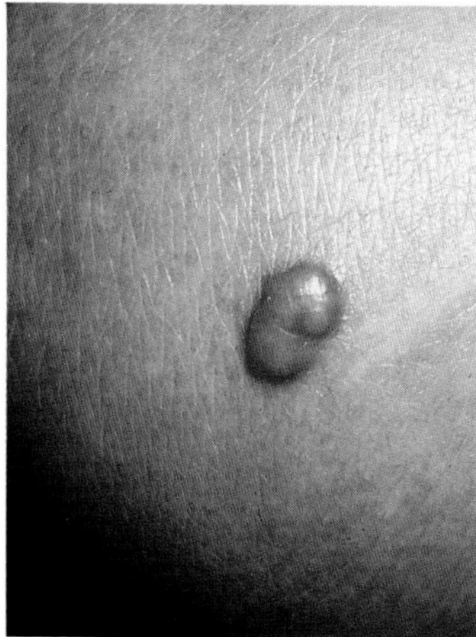

Fig. 67 Cutaneous sarcoidosis.

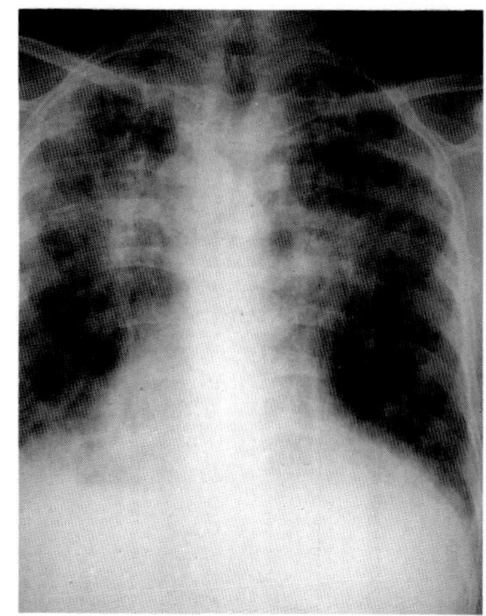

Fig. 68 Chronic pulmonary sarcoidosis—fibrosis of middle zones of both lungs.

Table 3 **Possible clinical features of chronic sarcoidosis**

Pulmonary
Bronchial inflammation
Lung fibrosis
Hilar lymphadenopathy

Skin
Erythema nodosum
Lupus pernio (nodules)

Eyes
Uveitis
Lacrimal gland enlargement
Keratoconjunctivitis sicca

Skeletal
Bone cysts
Arthritis
Hypercalcaemia

CNS
Focal signs
VII nerve palsy

Gut
Hepatosplenomegaly

Nose
Chronic rhinitis

Mouth
Non-specific deposits (e.g. gingivae)
Xerostomia
Parotid enlargement

Cardiac
Conductive defects

Table 4 **Causes of pneumonia**

Viral infection
Respiratory syncytial virus
Adenovirus
Influenza A
Cytomegalovirus (CMV) (pneumonia can develop in severe immunodeficiency)

Bacterial infection
Streptococcus pneumoniae (causes a lobar pneumonia)
Haemophilus influenzae
Mycobacterium tuberculosis
Mycoplasma pneumoniae
Chlamydia psittaci (psittacosis)
Staphylococcus aureus
Coxiella burnetti (Q fever)
Legionella pneumophila (Legionnaire's disease)
Klebsiella pneumoniae
Pseudomonas æruginosa

Protozoal infection
Pneumocystis carinii

Fungal infection
Aspergillus fumigatus

Chemical pneumonia
Aspiration of gastric contents (Mendelson syndrome), usually during periods of reduced consciousness or as a result of abnormal oesophageal structure or function

Radiation pneumonia
Radiation to the lungs can produce a localized inflammation

Allergic reactions
Allergic (type I) reactions to *Aspergillus fumigatus* may produce an eosinophilic pneumonia

Tuberculosis (TB)

Aetiology and epidemiology

Mycobacterium tuberculosis or *atypical* mycobacteria; common in the Third World, HIV disease, alcoholics and those of no fixed abode.

Pathology

Transmitted by droplets mainly. Caseating granulomas with later fibrosis and calcification. Dissemination via bloodstream causes widespread (miliary) infection.

Clinical features

Mostly asymptomatic infection but may cause:

- *enlarged cervical lymph nodes*—scrofula (Fig. 71)
- *pulmonary TB*—malaise, tiredness, anorexia, weight loss, chronic cough and haemoptysis
- *gastrointestinal disease*—oral ulcers, obstruction, perforation (Fig. 72) or peritonitis
- *genito-urinary disease*—various manifestations
- *CNS disease*—meningitis, encephalitis, cerebral abscess
- *skeletal disease*—osteomyelitis, abscesses, arthritis
- *cutaneous nodules*—lupus vulgaris
- *cardiovascular disease*—pericarditis
- *endocrine dysfunction*—adrenocortical failure.

Investigations

- Sputum, bronchial or gastric lavage or biopsy—culture and stain for acid-fast bacilli.
- Rapid or excessive Heaf or Mantoux reaction (unless immunocompromised).
- Chest radiograph.

Prevention

Bacille Calmette-Guérin (BCG) vaccine at 6 weeks for at-risk children; or at 13 years for others.

Management

Combination drugs, e.g. rifampicin plus isoniazid plus pyrazinamide with or without ethambutol for 6–9 months. Multidrug resistance can arise in some patient groups.

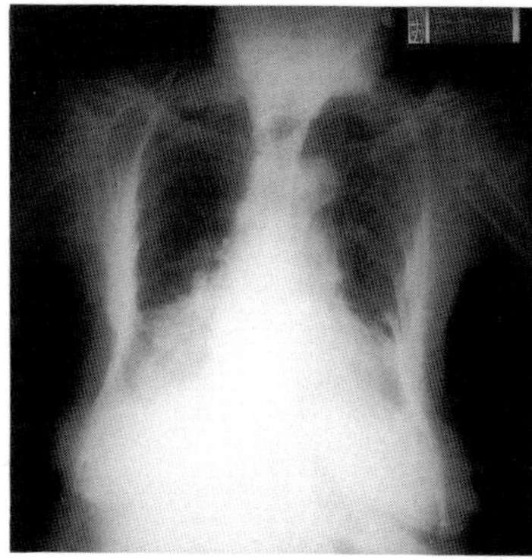

Fig. 69 Bilateral lower zone pneumonia.

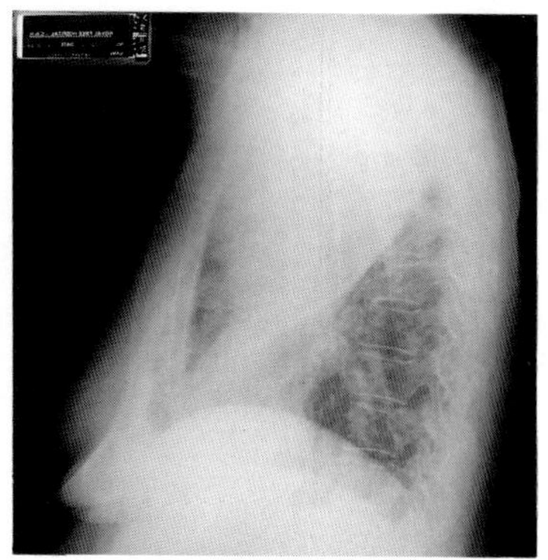

Fig. 70 Pneumonia of lower zones.

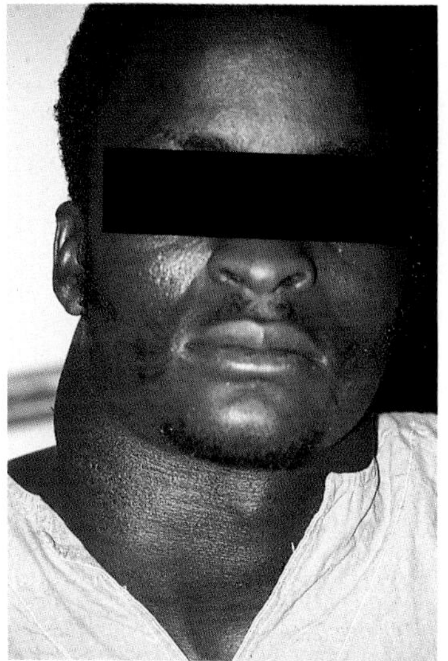

Fig. 71 Cervical lymph node enlargement in tuberculosis.

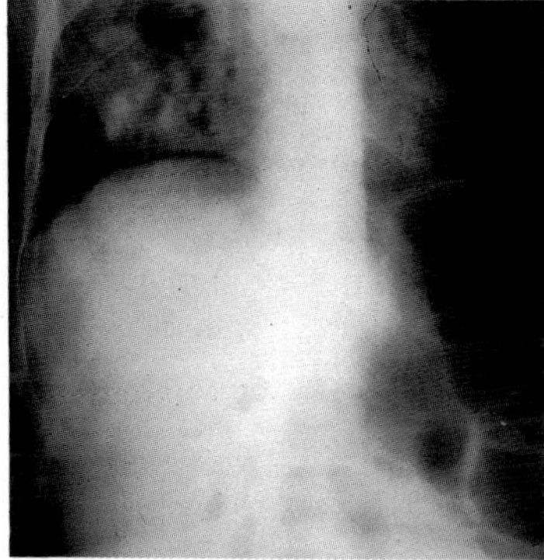

Fig. 72 Cavitation, calcification and fibrosis of lungs and ileal perforation in TB.

Bronchial carcinoma (lung cancer)

Epidemiology Most common cancer in the developed world.

Aetiology Cigarette smoking mainly (Fig. 73).

Pathology Usually squamous cell carcinoma; metastasizes to brain, bones and liver mainly.

Clinical features Cough and chest pain with or without haemoptysis (Table 5). There may also be: pneumonia; dyspnoea; hoarseness (infiltration of recurrent laryngeal nerve); dysphagia (infiltration of oesophagus); superior vena caval obstruction; Horner syndrome (ipsilateral loss of facial sweating, constricted pupil, ptosis and enophthalmos). *Metastatic disease* affects liver, kidney, bone and brain. *Non-metastatic extrapulmonary symptoms* such as acanthosis nigricans (Fig. 74) can also occur.

Investigations

- Chest radiograph—discrete opacity, hilar lymph node enlargement and consolidation.
- Sputum cytology.
- CT—can delineate tumour.
- Bronchoscopy—collection of bronchial washings and biopsy.
- Transthoracic fine-needle aspiration or thoracotomy may be needed for biopsy.

Management

- *Surgery*—often curative for early stage disease.
- *Radiotherapy*—an adjunct to surgery, or palliation.
- *Chemotherapy*—can benefit some tumours, e.g. small cell (oat cell) carcinoma.

Prognosis Poor, 5–10% survival at 5 years.

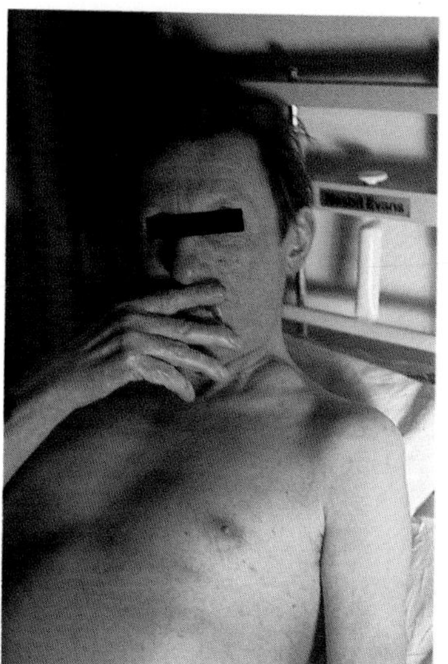

Fig. 73 Bronchial carcinoma: smoking, jaundice, clubbing and lymphadenopathy.

Table 5 **Causes of haemoptysis (blood-stained sputum)**

Pulmonary
Bronchial carcinoma (and other tumours)
TB or aspergillosis
Pneumonia
Pulmonary embolism, infarction
Bronchiectasis
Foreign body
Chronic bronchitis (uncommon)
Trauma
Goodpasture syndrome (uncommon vasculitis)

Other
Mitral stenosis (e.g. due to rupture of bronchopulmonary anastomoses)

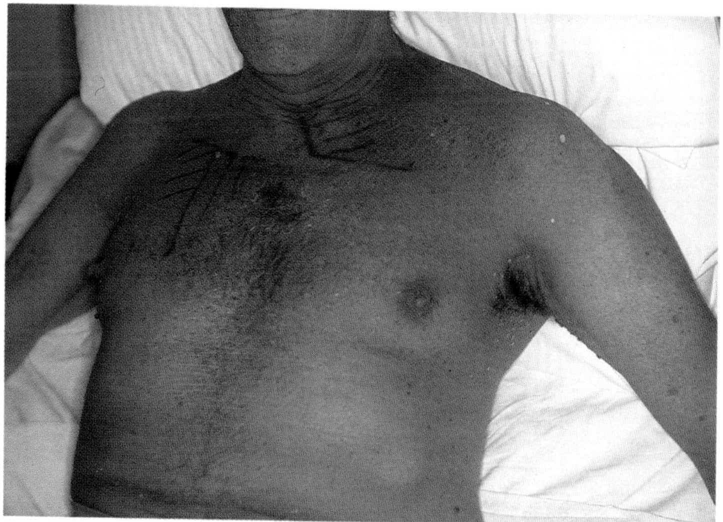

Fig. 74 Acanthosis nigricans in bronchial carcinoma.

5 / Haematological disease

Anaemia

Definition Decreased haemoglobin (Hb) concentration for age and gender of patient.

Aetiology Decreased red cell production (e.g. deficiency of haematinics or marrow failure); or excess red cell breakdown (e.g. haemolytic anaemia); or red cell loss (e.g. gastrointestinal, genitourinary or uterine bleeding).

Classification *Microcytic anaemia:* iron deficiency anaemia or thalassaemia.

Megaloblastic anaemia: vitamin B_{12} or folate deficiency.

Haemolytic anaemia: particularly sickle cell disease (Table 6).

Aplastic anaemia: usually viral or idiopathic.

Clinical features Pallor, breathlessness, angina, claudication, palpitations, tachycardia, ankle oedema.

Iron deficiency anaemia

Aetiology Inadequate diet (e.g. vegetarians), poor absorption (post-gastrectomy), excess utilization (haemolytic states) or excess loss (the most common cause).

Clinical features As for anaemia (above) plus sometimes angular stomatitis, oral ulcers, depapillated tongue (Fig. 75), koilonychia (i.e. spoon-shaped brittle nails, Fig. 76), hair loss.

Investigations Blood—decreased Hb, mean corpuscular volume (MCV) (i.e. microcytosis), packed cell volume (PCV) and mean corpuscular haemoglobin (MCH) (i.e. hypochromic); anisocytosis and poikilocytosis; reduced serum ferritin.

Management Investigate and manage underlying cause; iron supplements.

Table 6 **Causes of haemolytic anaemia**

Type	Cause
Congenital	Haemoglobinopathies: thalassaemias, sickle cell disease Membrane defects: hereditary spherocytosis, hereditary elliptocytosis Enzymic defects: glucose-6-phosphatase deficiency, pyruvate kinase deficiency
Acquired	Autoimmune destruction: systemic lupus erythematosus (IgG), rheumatoid arthritis (IgG), mycoplasma infection (IgM) Infection: malaria Drugs: aspirin and other non-steroidal anti-inflammatory drugs Mechanical destruction: prosthetic or infected heart valves, burns Hypersplenism: neoplasms leukaemias, lymphomas

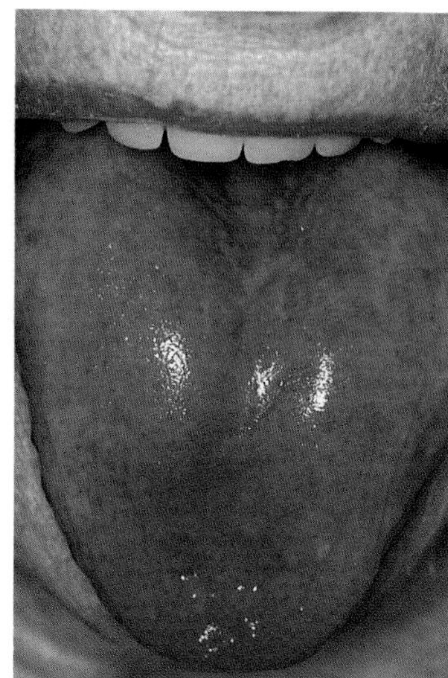

Fig. 75 Glossitis in anaemia.

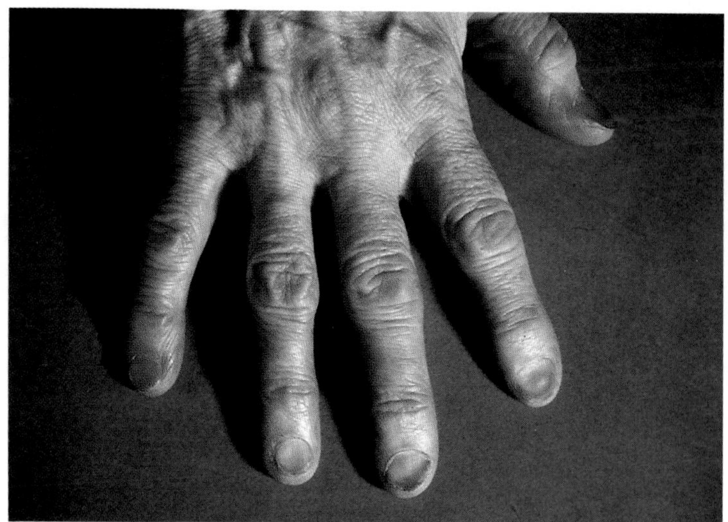

Fig. 76 Koilonychia in iron deficiency anaemia.

Vitamin B_{12} deficiency anaemia

Aetiology

Usually pernicious anaemia (i.e. autoantibody against gastric parietal cells (Fig. 77), post-gastrectomy, small bowel disease or resection. Vegans are at risk.

Clinical features

The general features of anaemia (p. 53), plus sometimes lemon-tinged skin (hyperbilirubinaemia), angular stomatitis, red-beefy tongue, mouth ulcers, peripheral neuropathy and subacute combined degeneration, changes in mood, dementia.

Investigations

- Blood—reduced Hb and RBC levels, MCV raised (macrocytosis), poikilocytosis, increased nuclear segmentation of neutrophils.
- Bone marrow—megaloblastosis.
- Reduced serum vitamin B_{12}.
- Possibly Schilling test positive.
- Parietal cell antibodies antibodies in pernicious anaemia.

Management

Manage underlying cause. Vitamin B_{12} (hydroxycobalamin) injections are needed for life.

Folic acid deficiency

Aetiology

Usually inadequate dietary folic acid.

Clinical features

The general features of anaemia (p. 53) plus sometimes oral and cutaneous ulceration (Figs 78 & 79), angular stomatitis and sore tongue.

Investigations

- Blood—reduced Hb, raised MCV.
- Reduced red-cell folate.
- Normal serum vitamin B_{12} levels.

Management

Manage underlying cause. Treat with folic acid—oral supplements.

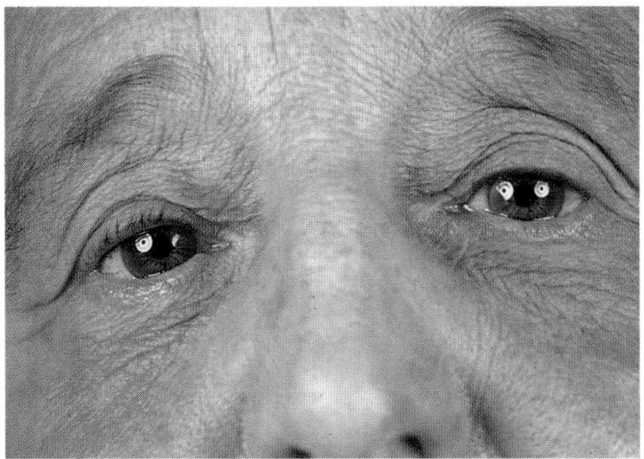

Fig. 77 Pernicious anaemia: more common in Scandinavians (blonde and blue-eyed).

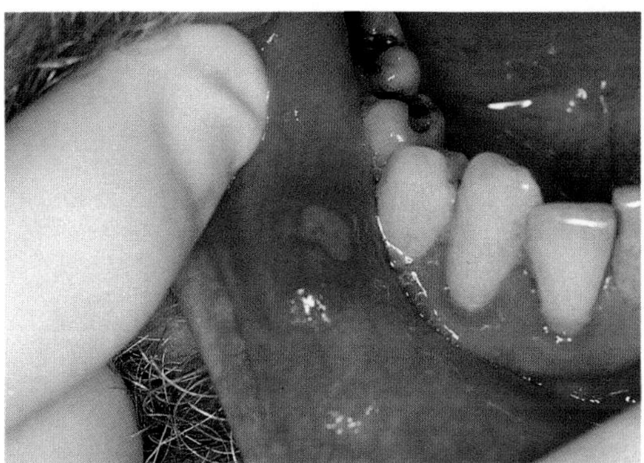

Fig. 78 Oral ulceration in folic acid deficiency.

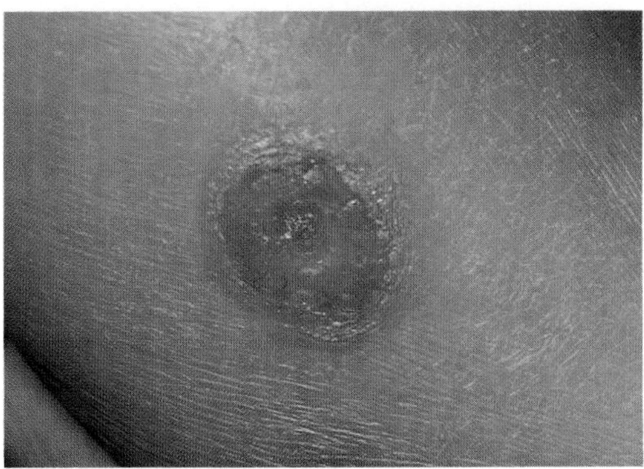

Fig. 79 Cutaneous ulceration in folic acid deficiency.

Thalassaemia

Definition and epidemiology

Defect in haemoglobin chain number. Autosomal recessive inheritance, predominantly in people from the Mediterranean littoral.

Clinical features

Anaemia, excess bone marrow production (reduced stature, frontal bossing, maxillary hyperplasia) and excess breakdown of red blood cells (hepatosplenomegaly, gallstones).

Investigations

- Microcytic hypochromic anaemia.
- Haemoglobin electrophoresis—defines defect.
- Possibly elevated serum ferritin—from transfusions.
- Radiographs—expansion of marrow and cortical thinning, 'hair on end' appearance of skull (Fig. 80).

Management

Transfusions; folic acid; remove excess iron with desferrioxamine.

Sickle cell disease

Definition and epidemiology

Defect in haemoglobin chain structure. Autosomal dominant inheritance, mainly in African descendants. Homozygote sickle cell disease has *anaemia*; the heterozygote has *sickle cell trait*—only mild haemolysis.

Clinical features

Haemolytic anaemia, infections, painful swellings of hands (Fig. 81) and feet, haematuria, renal papillary necrosis, leg ulcers, splenic infarction, retinopathy, jaundice, gallstones and hepatomegaly. *Painful crises* affect chest, bone, or spleen and are precipitated by cold, hypoxia, infection, dehydration or exercise. *Aplastic crises* are due to parvovirus infection.

Investigations

Sickle cell screen (SickleDex); blood film; haemoglobin level and electrophoresis.

Treatment

Folic acid; prevent crises, avoid complications; blood transfusion in severe anaemia.

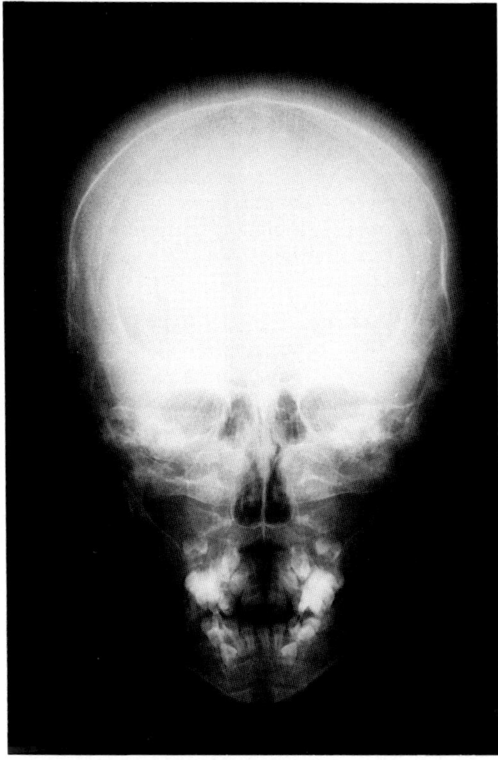

Fig. 80 'Hair on end' appearance of tables of skull in thalassaemia major.

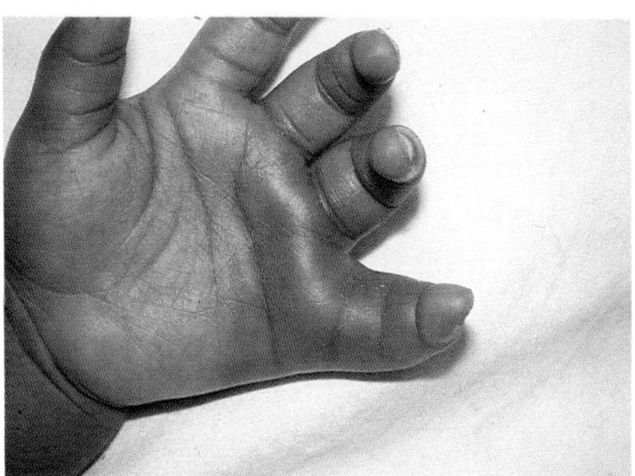

Fig. 81 Dactylitis secondary to osteomyelitis in sickle cell disease.

Acute leukaemias

Definition

Neoplastic lymphoblasts or myeloblasts.

Aetiology

Associations with:
- myeloproliferative disorders or immunodeficiency
- chromosomal anomalies (e.g. trisomy 21, Fanconi's anaemia)
- exposure to benzene and possibly viruses
- association with radiation exposure is controversial.

Clinical features

Anaemia, neutropenia (liability to infections, Fig. 82) and thrombocytopenia (e.g. purpura, Fig. 83). Lymphadenopathy, bone pain, hepatosplenomegaly and oral ulcers also occur.

Investigations

- Blood—normal or abnormal white cell count, and blasts.
- Marrow biopsy—abnormal blasts.

Management

- Cytotoxics plus corticosteroids.
- CNS irradiation and intrathecal chemotherapy.
- Bone marrow transplantation.

Prognosis

Childhood acute lymphoblastic leukaemia has a 70% 5-year survival.
Acute myeloid leukaemia has a 20% 5-year survival rate.

Chronic lymphocytic leukaemia

Epidemiology

Most common leukaemia. Occurs in middle to late life.

Clinical features

Often asymptomatic, but may cause lymphadenopathy, splenomegaly, viral and fungal infection, and skin infiltration.

Investigations

White blood cell count—raised lymphocytes.

Management

- Chlorambucil, cyclophosphamide in early symptomatic disease.
- Palliative radiotherapy.

Prognosis

Survival can be as long as 12–14 years.

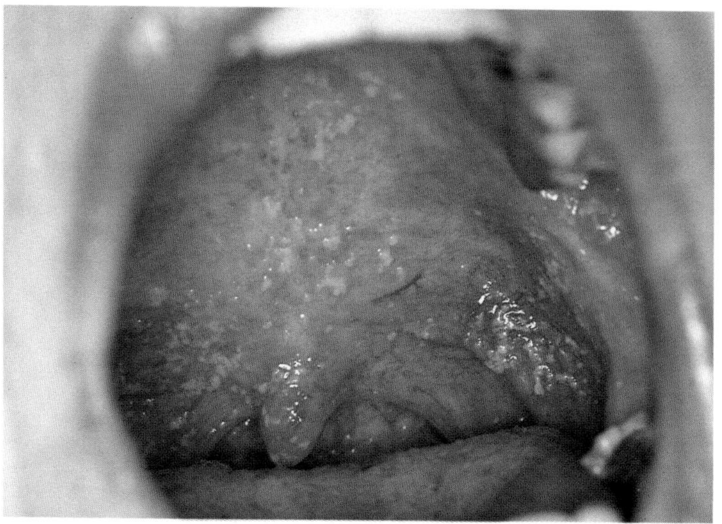

Fig. 82 Oral candidosis in acute lymphoblastic leukaemia.

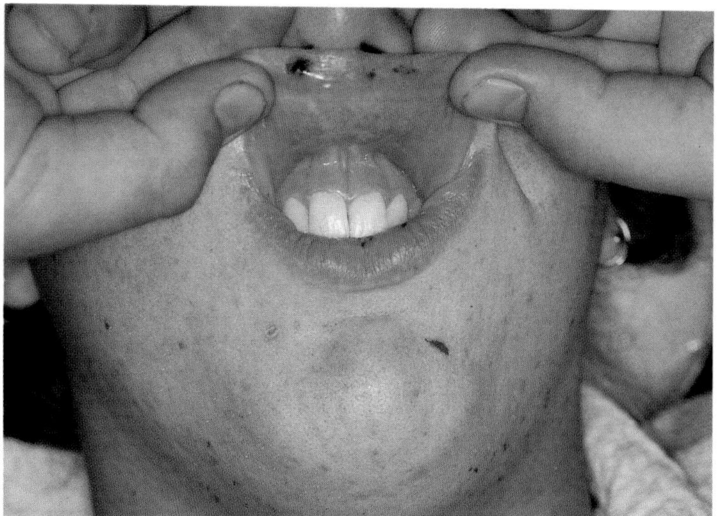

Fig. 83 Oral purpura in late chronic lymphocytic leukaemia.

Chronic myeloid leukaemia

Aetiology

95% of those affected have the Philadelphia chromosome.

Clinical features

Asymptomatic; or anaemia, splenomegaly (Fig. 84) causing abdominal pain, gout, thrombocytopenia.

Investigations

- Blood—raised white cell count, neutrophilia, basophilia, anaemia, variable platelet count.
- Marrow—granulocytic hyperplasia.

Management

Symptomatic (e.g. splenectomy, correct anaemias), chemotherapy.

Prognosis

Can progress to acute leukaemia, invariably fatal within 4 years.

Multiple myeloma (myelomatosis)

Definition and pathology

Neoplastic plasma cells in bone with progressive bone marrow failure, immunodeficiency and monoclonal gammopathy (i.e. paraprotein—usually IgG). Bence-Jones protein (immunoglobulin light chains) present in blood and urine.

Clinical features

Anaemia, neutropenia and thrombocytopenia; bone pain and fractures; focal neurological signs; renal failure; hyperviscosity (e.g. headache, blurred vision, mucosal bleeding).

Investigations

- Blood—plasma cells, anaemia, thrombocytopenia, raised ESR, hypercalcaemia, hyperuricaemia.
- Radiographs—radiolucencies (Fig. 85), pathological fractures.
- Serum electrophoresis—raised gammaglobulins (M band).
- Bence-Jones protein in urine.

Management

Chemotherapy and palliative radiotherapy for bone pain.

Prognosis

Most die within 3 years. Multiple myeloma predisposes to amyloidosis.

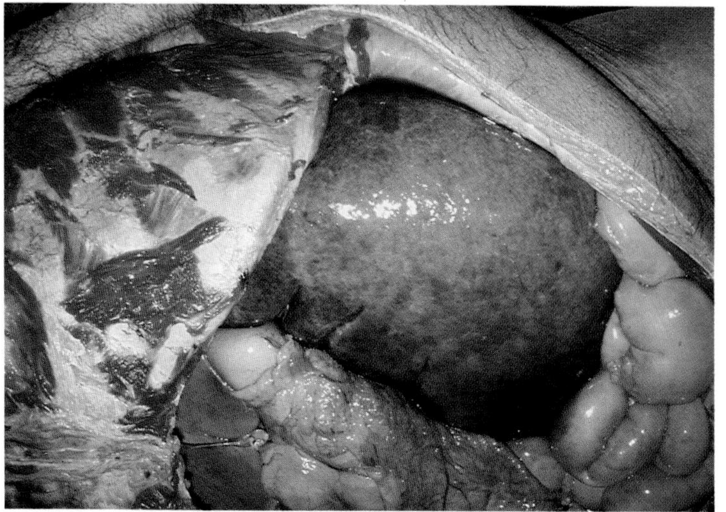

Fig. 84 Splenomegaly in chronic myeloid leukaemia.

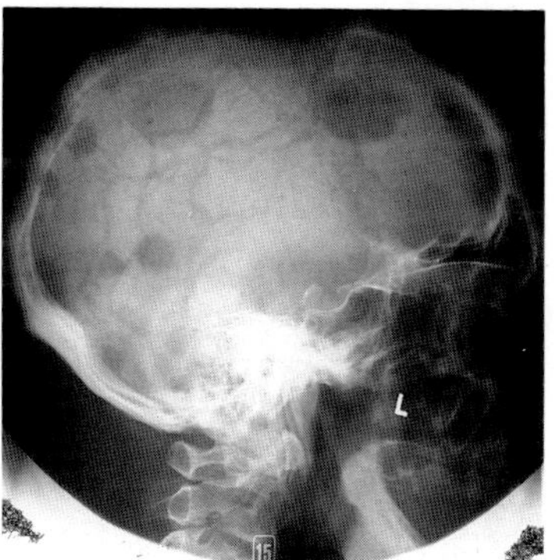

Fig. 85 'Pepper pot' skull radiograph in multiple myeloma.

Hodgkin's disease

Definition

Tumour with neoplastic cells of monocyte lineage (Reed–Sternberg cells).

Pathology

Variable histology (e.g. lymphocyte predominant, mixed cellularity, nodular sclerosing, lymphocyte depleted). Typically affects lymphoid tissue and spreads via lymphatics.

Clinical features

Lymphadenopathy (typically cervical, Fig. 86), hepatomegaly and splenomegaly; night sweats, weight loss and pyrexia ('B' symptoms).

Investigations

- Lymph node biopsy.
- Biochemistry—raised serum calcium and uric acid, abnormal liver function test (LFT).
- Chest radiography and thoracoabdominal CT/magnetic resonance imaging (MRI) for *staging*.

Management

Local radiotherapy for early disease. More extensive disease or 'B' symptoms necessitate cytotoxics and corticosteroids.

Prognosis

Over 90% long-term survival in early disease.

Non-Hodgkin's lymphoma

Definition

Tumour of neoplastic lymphocytes.

Pathology

Initially involves extralymphoid sites and spreads in an unpredictable manner (Fig. 87). There is an increasing incidence in immunodeficiency possibly reflecting some viral causes such as EBV.

Clinical features

Similar to Hodgkin's disease, but affected sites may not be contiguous. Abdominal involvement is common.

Investigations

As Hodgkin's disease.

Management

Radiotherapy plus chemotherapy.

Prognosis

Usually poorer than in Hodgkin's disease: 5-year survival up to 60–70%.

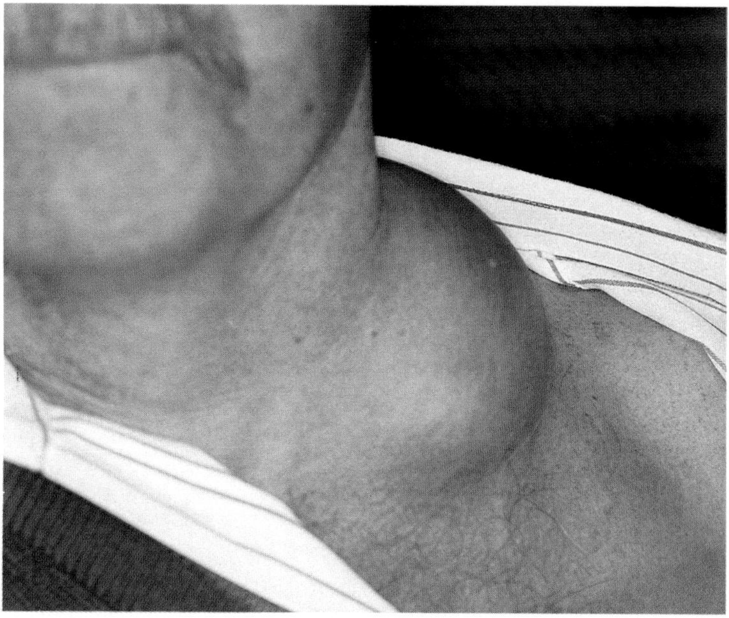

Fig. 86 Supraclavicular lymphadenopathy in Hodgkin's lymphoma.

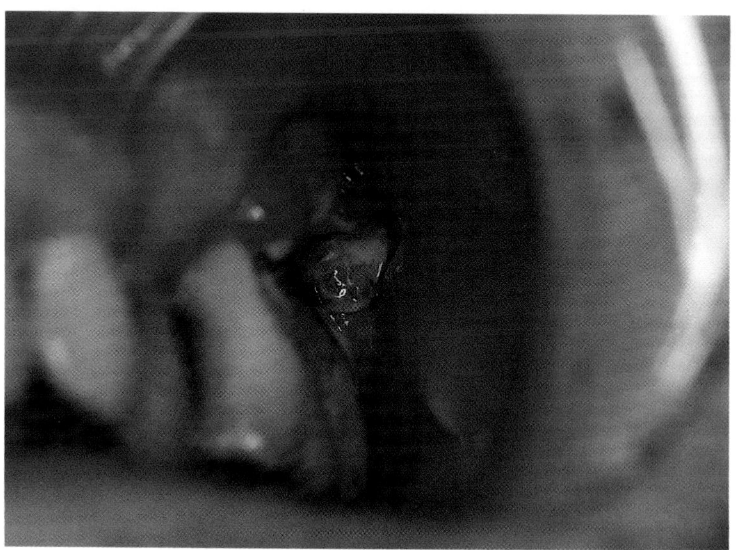

Fig. 87 Non-Hodgkin's lymphoma of the mouth in AIDS.

Thrombocytopenic purpura

Aetiology

Bone marrow suppression (e.g. leukaemia) or damage (e.g. cytotoxics); or platelet destruction or utilization (e.g. in autoimmune thrombocytopenia).

Clinical features

Purpura (Figs 88 & 89), epistaxis, menorrhagia.

Investigations

- Platelet and white cell count.
- Prolonged bleeding time.
- Normal coagulation tests.

Management

Manage underlying cause. Treat with platelet transfusions, corticosteroids, azathioprine and immunoglobulins.

Coagulation disorders

Aetiology

Hereditary: haemophilia A (reduced factor VIII—sex-linked recessive); haemophilia B (reduced factor IX—sex-linked recessive); and Von Willebrand's disease (*defective* factor VIII plus platelet defect—autosomal dominant).

Acquired: more common; usually due to defective synthesis of vitamin K-dependent factors (e.g. by anticoagulants).

Clinical features

Large, deep ecchymoses; general bleeding (Fig. 90) into joints (haemarthroses, Fig. 91) and body cavities (including intracranially). The patient may have blood-borne viral infections (e.g. HIV, HBV, HCV secondary to transfusions received prior to routine screening of blood donations).

Investigations

- Normal bleeding time, platelet numbers and function.
- Prolonged activated partial thromboplastin time (APTT) or prothrombin time (PT).
- Reduced levels of specific clotting factors.

Management

Blood clotting factor replacement, antifibrinolytics (e.g. tranexamic acid), desmopressin.

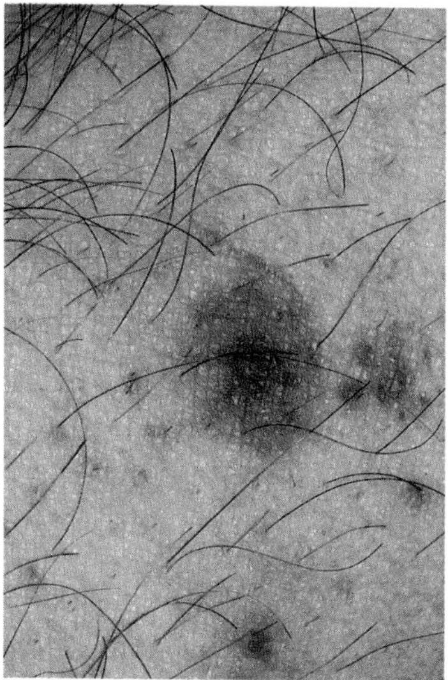

Fig. 88 Thrombocytopenic purpura.

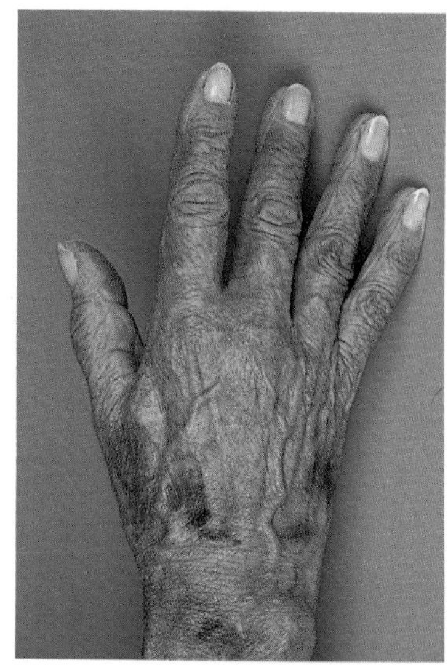

Fig. 89 Thrombocytopenic purpura.

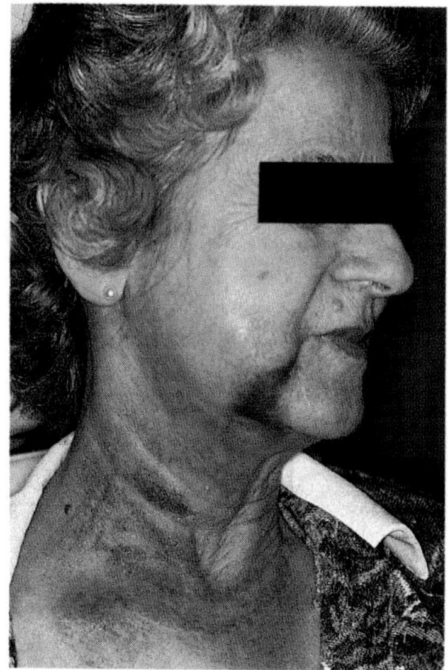

Fig. 90 Severe post-extraction bleeding in a coagulation disorder—rare nowadays.

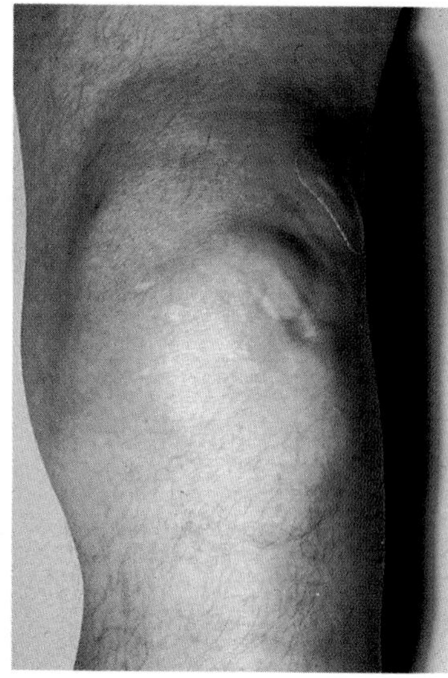

Fig. 91 Bleeding into joint spaces in haemophilia.

6 / Salivary gland disease

Pleomorphic adenoma

Pathology

Usually benign. Origin unclear but typically contains both epithelial and myxoid elements ('mixed salivary gland tumour').

Clinical features

Slow-growing swelling (Fig. 92). Facial palsy is very rare and may denote malignant change.

Investigations

CT or MRI can delineate extent of tumour. Ultrasound is occasionally useful. A needle biopsy may be indicated.

Management

Resection—recurs if incomplete. The prognosis is good.

Adenoid cystic carcinoma

Pathology

More commonly affects intraoral salivary glands. The tumour has a typical cribriform (cylindromatous) histological appearance and a tendency for perineural spread.

Clinical features

Slow-growing lump (Figs 93 & 94) that can ulcerate. Involvement of nerves can cause pain, paraesthesia, anaesthesia and palsies.

Investigation

CT or MRI may delineate lesion. Chest radiographs are needed to exclude metastases. A needle biopsy may be indicated.

Management

Radical resection *and* local radiotherapy. 60% 5-year survival.

Salivary calculus

Pathology

Obstruction of duct causes swelling. The condition typically affects the submandibular gland (Fig. 95).

Clinical features

Pain and swelling mainly at mealtimes.

Investigations

Radiography.

Management

Surgical removal or lithotripsy.

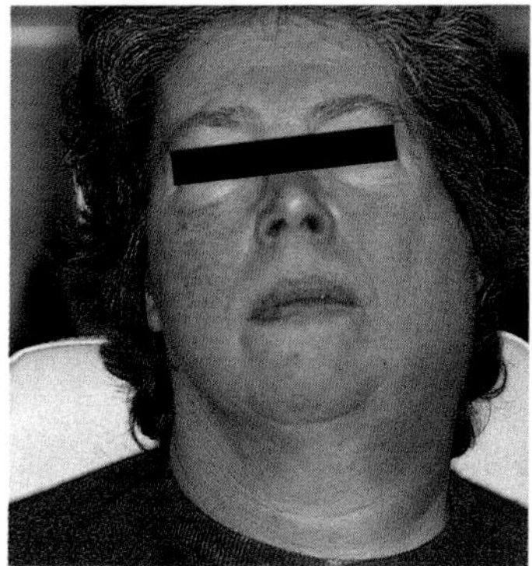

Fig. 92 Pleomorphic adenoma of left parotid gland.

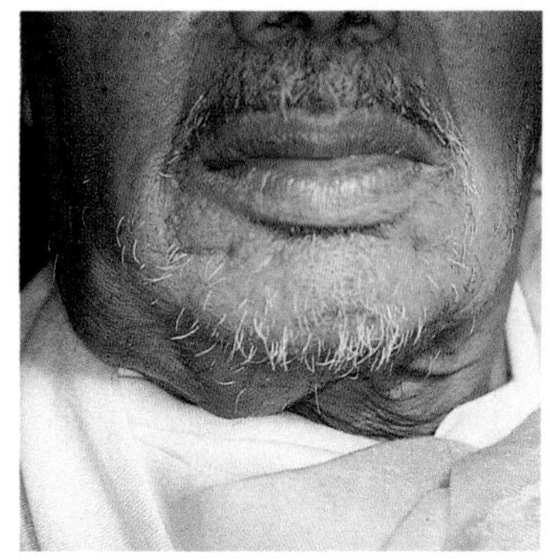

Fig. 93 Adenoid cystic carcinoma of right submandibular gland.

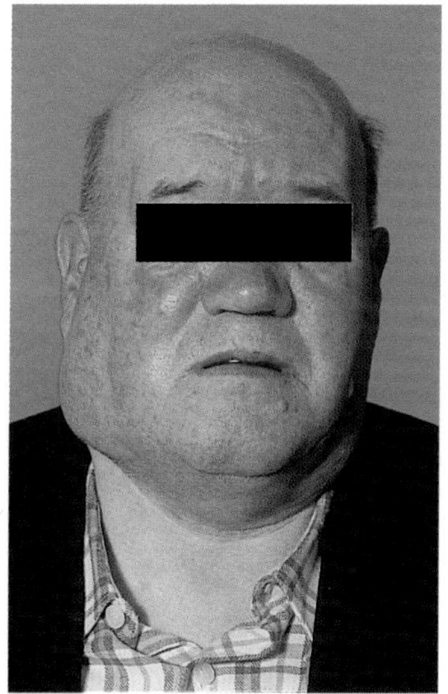

Fig. 94 Large acinic cell carcinoma of the parotid gland—another malignant tumour of the salivary glands.

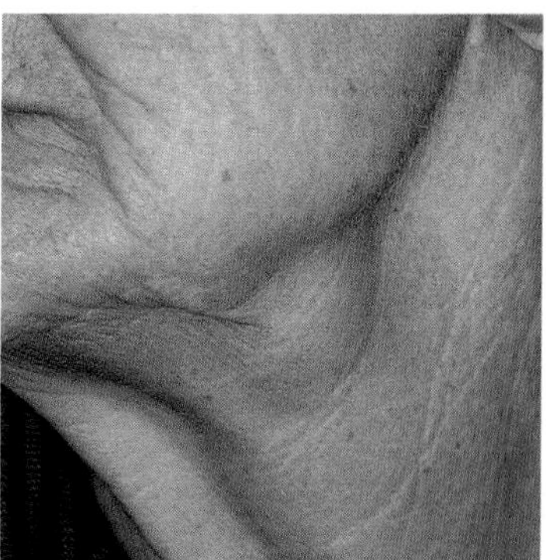

Fig. 95 Salivary swelling due to submandibular calculus.

7 / Neck masses

Clinical types (Table 7)

Lymphadenitis: mainly from infection in the head and neck occasionally mycobacterial (Fig. 96).

Sebaceous cyst: mobile superficial swelling which may have a punctum and can become infected.

Lipoma: soft, fluctuant, mobile swelling.

Furuncle: deep infection of contiguous hair follicles.

Ranula: cyst arising from retention of saliva in sublingual gland.

Epidermoid cyst: usually of congenital origin; occurs in submental area.

Thyroglossal cyst: characteristically presents as midline lump that moves on swallowing.

Goitre: see page 97.

Metastases from tumours in head and neck: from mouth, thyroid, oesophagus, larynx, pharynx and distant sites (Fig. 97).

Laryngocele: laryngeal mucosa herniates through thyrohyoid membrane—seen in some wind instrument players (Fig. 98).

Lymphoma: see page 63.

Branchial cyst: painless lump anterior to upper third of sternomastoid muscle. It is fluctuant, mobile, and can become infected.

Cystic hygroma: lymphangioma, usually in posterior triangle.

Carotid aneurysm: pulsatile mass in line of major blood vessels.

Submandibular gland disease: obstruction, infection or neoplasia.

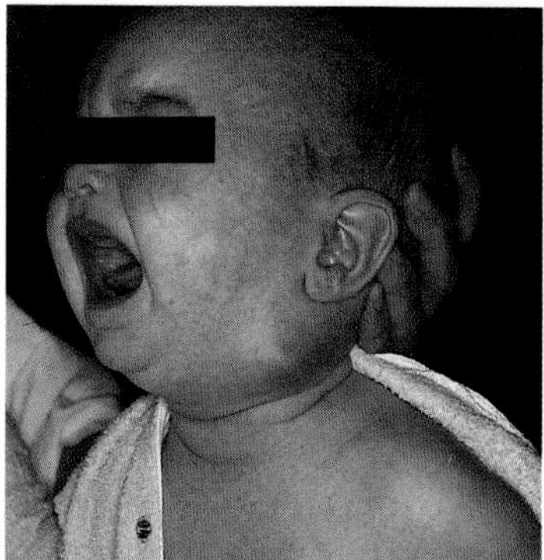

Fig. 96 Cervical lymphadenitis, note the redness and swelling.

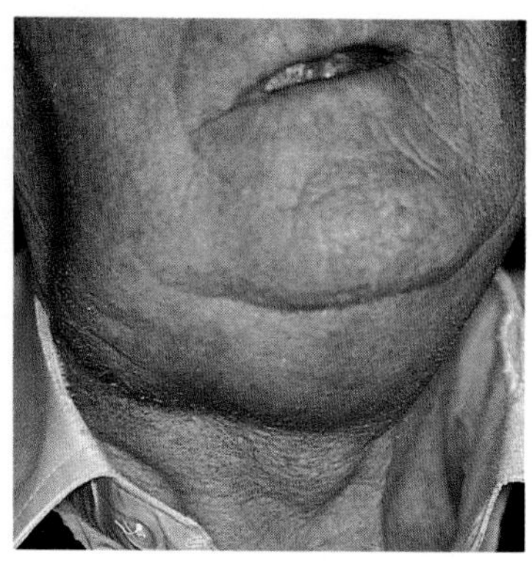

Fig. 97 Cervical lymphadenopathy due to oral squamous cell carcinoma.

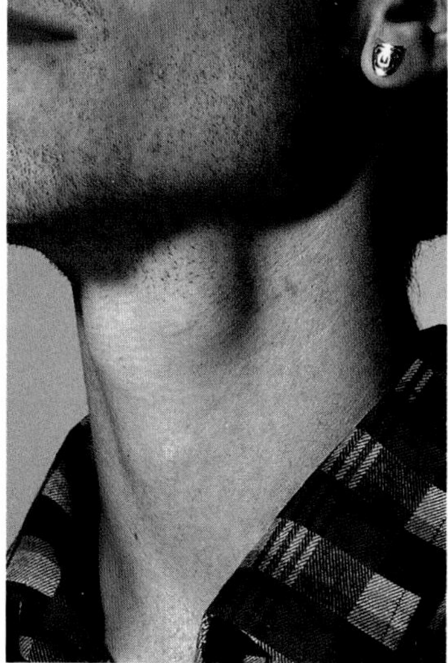

Fig. 98 Laryngocele.

Table 7 **Neck masses**

Location	Type
Superficial	Sebaceous cyst Neurofibroma Lipoma Carbuncle Furuncle
Deep	Plunging ranula Epidermoid cyst Thyroglossal cyst Goitre Neoplasia Laryngocele Pharyngeal pouch Cervical lymphadenopathy *Infection*: any local infection in head and neck, EBV, HIV, HSV, other viruses, syphilis, actinomycosis, TB, atypical mycobacterioses, cat-scratch disease, toxoplasmosis. *Neoplasia:* head and neck, gastric, bronchial, other secondaries, lymphomas (especially Hodgkin's), leukaemia *Others*: Sarcoidosis, cherubism Branchial cyst Sternomastoid tumour Cystic hygroma Carotid/subclavian aneurysm Carotid body tumour Salivary tumours

8 / Gastrointestinal disease

Dysphagia

Definition Difficulty in swallowing (painful or otherwise).

Aetiology Can have various causes (Table 8), such as oesophageal diverticulum (Fig. 99).

Clinical features Food 'sticks' in throat or chest, sometimes with regurgitation.

Investigations

- Barium swallow.
- Endoscopy and biopsies.
- Manometry—in motility disorders.

Management Treat underlying cause.

Oesophageal carcinoma

Epidemiology Common in China and parts of Africa.

Aetiology Carcinogens in diet, iron deficiency anaemia (Plummer–Vinson syndrome), alcohol, smoking, achalasia (Fig. 100), oesophageal metaplasia.

Pathology Usually squamous cell carcinoma (Fig. 101).

Clinical features Progressive dysphagia, with eventual difficulty in swallowing saliva resulting in coughing and aspiration into the lungs. Other features are haematemesis, weight loss, anorexia and lymphadenopathy.

Investigations

- Barium swallow (Fig. 102, p. 74).
- Oesophagoscopy and biopsy.
- CT/MRI can delineate lesion.

Management Surgery usually for lesions in lower oesophagus; radiotherapy, possibly adjuvant chemotherapy.

Prognosis Appalling: 2% survival at 5 years.

Table 8 **Causes of dysphagia**

Painful oral lesions **Pharyngeal pouches** **Oral and pharyngeal neoplasms** **Neuromuscular disease** Myasthenia gravis, bulbar palsy (i.e. defect at level of IX, X, XI, XII nuclei), pseudobulbar palsy **Defective oesophageal motility** Scleroderma Achalasia (defective relaxation in lower oesophagus), diffuse oesophageal spasm **Lesions of oesophagus** Foreign body, strictures (e.g. due to reflux, acids/alkalis or neoplasia)	**Lesion of adjacent structures** Hilar lymph node enlargement, goitre, bronchial carcinoma, enlarged left atrium (rare) **Psychogenic** Globus syndrome (sometimes incorrectly termed 'globus hystericus')—sensation of a lump in the throat, that does not actually interfere with swallowing. The diagnosis can only be made after detailed exclusion of organic disease.

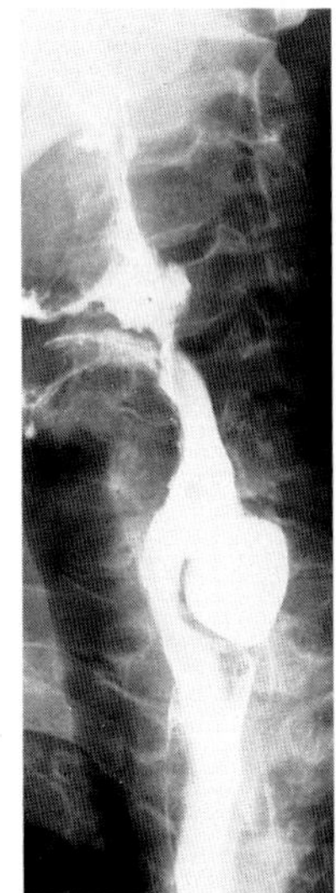

Fig. 99 Pharyngeal pouch.

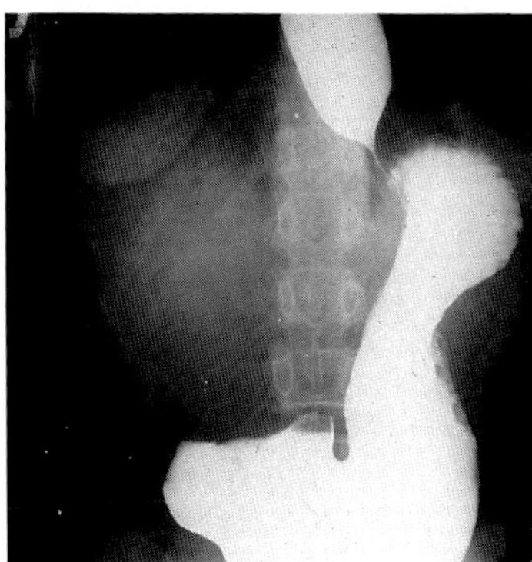

Fig. 100 Achalasia of the distal oesophagus.

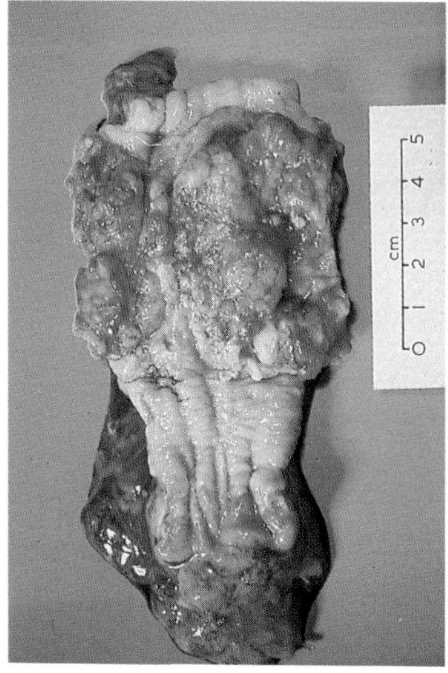

Fig. 101 Postmortem oesophageal squamous cell carcinoma.

Hiatus hernia

Definition

Stomach herniates (usually slides) through diaphragm into thorax (Fig. 103).

Aetiology

Raised intra-abdominal pressure (e.g. obesity), smoking and anticholinergic drugs predispose. Occasionally the condition is congenital.

Clinical features

Retrosternal pain, typically on lying or bending and relieved by antacids. Food may regurgitate.

Investigations

Barium swallow, oesophagoscopy, manometry.

Management

- Correct associated factors.
- Antacids (with or without alginates).
- H_2 blockers (ranitidine); proton pump inhibitors, e.g. omeprazole.
- Surgery—rarely.

Complications

Stricture, haematemesis, anaemia.

Gastritis

Definition

Inflamed gastric mucosa.

Pathology

Erosive: due to non-steroidal anti-inflammatory drugs (NSAIDs) or stress.

Non-erosive: autoimmune, often associated with pernicious anaemia (Type A) or with *Helicobacter pylori* infection (Type B).

Clinical features

Often asymptomatic, but can cause epigastric pain, bloating or nausea.

Investigations

- Barium meal.
- Endoscopy and biopsy and/or culture for *H. pylori.*
- *H. pylori* antibodies.
- Anti-parietal cell antibodies.
- Breath tests.

Management

- *Erosive*—antacids and avoid NSAIDs.
- *Type A disease*—nil unless pernicious anaemia evident.
- *Type B disease*—bismuth, amoxycillin or metronidazole.

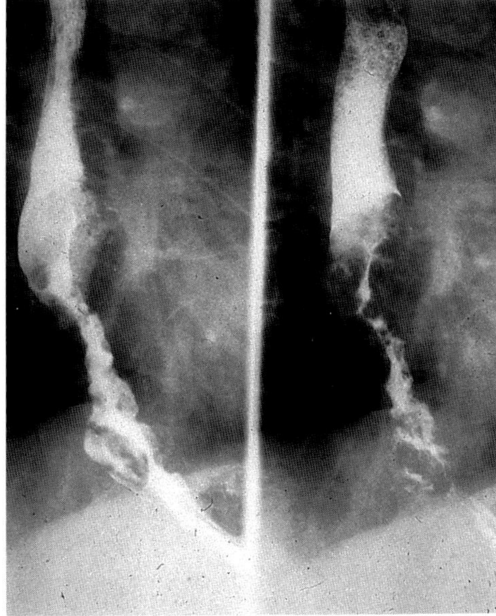

Fig. 102 Barium swallow showing oesophageal carcinoma.

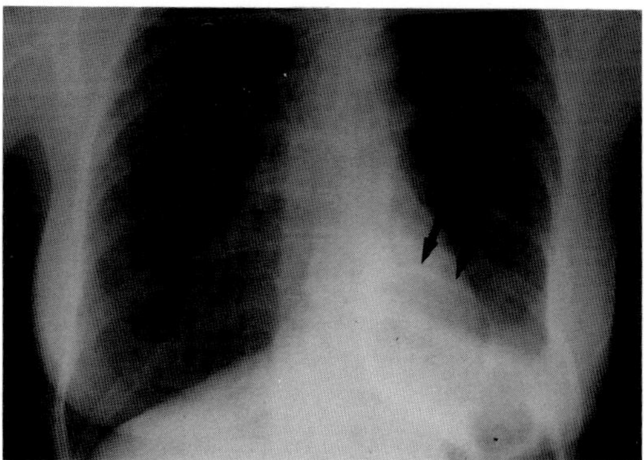

Fig. 103 Gas bubble above left hemidiaphragm: hiatus hernia.

Peptic ulceration

Definition

Ulcer of stomach or duodenum.

Aetiology

Reduced mucus, chronic gastritis, biliary reflux and mucosal ischaemia may be important in gastric ulcers. Duodenal ulceration is associated with excess acid and pepsinogen. *H. pylori* may be of significance. NSAIDs, smoking, blood group O and a family history of peptic ulceration are important in both, but stress appears *not* to be a major factor.

Clinical features

Duodenal ulcer: epigastric pain when hungry. Condition may cause haemorrhage, obstruction (due to pyloric stenosis) or perforation.

Gastric ulcer (Fig. 104): pain mainly after eating, and bleeding with anaemia. Perforation is unlikely.

Investigations

- Barium studies (Fig. 105).
- Endoscopy and biopsy.
- Gastric secretion rates—rarely of value.

Management

- Bed rest.
- Stop smoking.
- Reduce alcohol consumption.
- Avoid dietary precipitants.
- Drugs—autibiotics if *H. pylori,* antacids; H_2 blockers (ranitidine/cimetidine); proton pump inhibitor, e.g. omeprazole; anticholinergics (pirenzepine); prostaglandin E analogue (misoprostol). *Avoid* NSAIDs and corticosteroids.
- Surgery for recalcitrant disease, severe haemorrhage, perforation or obstruction.

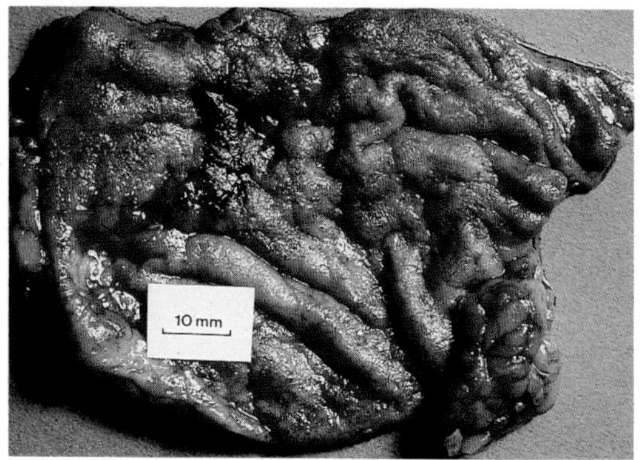

Fig. 104 Gastric ulceration: postmortem specimen.

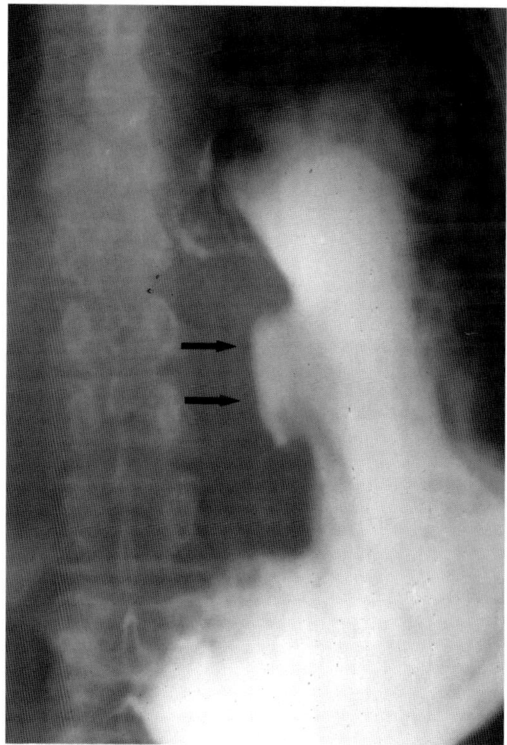

Fig. 105 Barium meal: large ulcer on lesser curve of stomach.

Gastric carcinoma

Aetiology

Achlorhydria, pernicious anaemia, chronic ulceration, polyps, blood group A, nitrates in diet, alcohol, spicy foods, dietary carcinogens, smoking.

Pathology

Usually adenocarcinoma.

Clinical features

Epigastric pain and mass, anorexia, nausea, weight loss, anaemia (Fig. 106). Dysphagia may occur if the fundus is involved. Other features are haematemesis (uncommon), supraclavicular lymphadenopathy (Troisier's sign—rare), liver enlargement and other metastatic disease.

Investigations

- Barium meal.
- Endoscopy and biopsy.

Management

Partial gastrectomy or celestin tube as palliation.

Prognosis

Poor: 10% survival at 5 years.

Haematemesis

Aetiology

Table 9.

Investigations

Endoscopy.

Management

Resuscitate. Stop profuse bleeding (e.g. via endoscopic cautery, laser therapy, local injection of vasoconstrictor), or close via surgery.

Bleeding from rectum

Aetiology

Table 10.

Clinical features

If the bleeding is high in the gut, the stools will be black and tarry (melaena). Bleeding from the lower gut may produce stools with bloody streaks or frank blood.

Investigations

GI endoscopy, colonoscopy, proctosigmoidoscopy.

Management

Manage underlying cause.

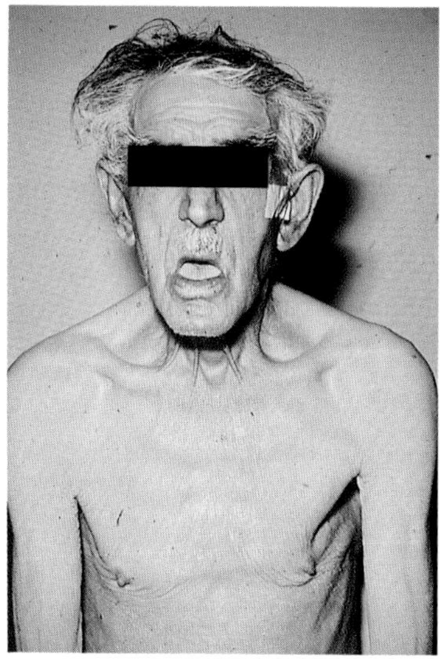

Fig. 106 Profound cachexia and jaundice due to gastric carcinoma.

Table 9 **Causes of haematemesis (vomiting of blood)***

Oesophageal
Reflux oesophagitis
Varices in hepatic cirrhosis
Mallory–Weiss syndrome (tear after vomiting)
Cancer
Aortic aneurysm (rare)

Gastric
Gastritis (e.g. alcohol, NSAIDs)
Erosion
Ulceration
Cancer

Duodenal
Ulceration

Other
Bleeding tendency
Some hereditary connective tissue disorders (rare)

**Can also occur secondary to epistaxis or severe post-dental extraction bleeding*

Table 10 **Causes of bleeding from rectum**

Anal canal
Haemorrhoids (Fig. 107)
Fissures
Fistulae

Large intestine
Inflammatory bowel disease
Angiodysplasia
Adenomatous polyps
Carcinoma
Ischaemic colitis
Intussusception
Diverticulitis

Small intestine
Meckel's diverticulum
Arteriovenous fistula

Other
Bleeding tendency
Infection

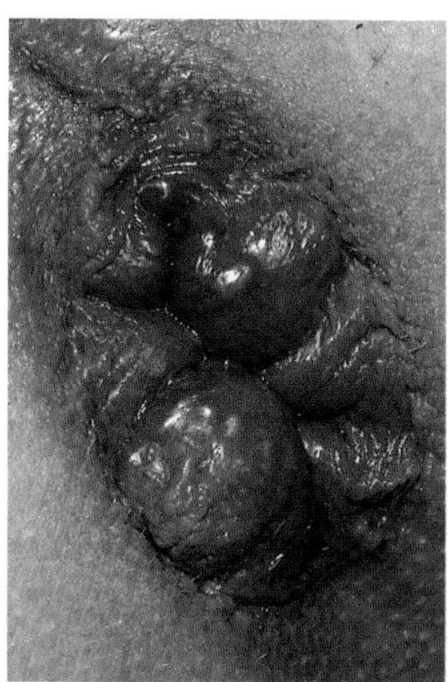

Fig. 107 Haemorrhoids (piles): the most common cause of rectal bleeding.

Malabsorption

Aetiology

Table 11.

Clinical features

Failure to thrive, diarrhoea/steatorrhoea, abdominal pain, weight loss and evidence of nutritional deficiencies, e.g. sore mouth, angular cheilitis or ulcers. The condition may be subclinical.

Investigations

- Full blood picture; serum calcium, iron, vitamin B_{12}, albumin and red cell folate assays.
- Faecal fats (raised) or $^{14}CO_2$ breath analysis.
- Antireticulin antibodies, and villous atrophy on small bowel biopsy in coeliac disease.

Management

Treat cause and correct nutritional abnormalities. A gluten-free diet is required for coeliac disease.

Gallstones

Aetiology

- *Cholesterol stones* (most common)—middle age, obesity, contraceptive pill, gut disease (e.g. Crohn's).
- *Bile pigment stones*—gallbladder infection, chronic bile obstruction, haemolytic states and cirrhosis.

Symptoms

Symptomless; painless jaundice (Fig. 108); or epigastric pain with fatty foods. Infection (acute cholecystitis) produces epigastric pain, nausea, vomiting, pyrexia, flatulence, shallow breathing, and guarding.

Investigations

Plain radiographs (Fig. 109), or ultrasound. Radiolucent stones are also delineated by transhepatic cholangiography or more commonly endoscopic retrograde cholangiopancreatography (ERCP).

Management

- Symptomless stones—cholecystectomy.
- *Acute cholecystitis*—bed rest, analgesia, i.v. fluids and antibiotics; then cholecystectomy.
- *Duct stones*—endoscopic removal or cholecystectomy with or without exploration of duct.

Complications

Perforation and peritonitis.

Table 11 **Causes of malabsorption**

Mucosal disease	Inadequate supply of bile acids
Coeliac disease (gluten sensitive enteropathy)*	Intestinal resection*
Tropical sprue	Irradiation damage
Giardiasis	Hepatocellular damage*
Lymphoma	Biliary obstruction*
Hypogammaglobulinaemia	Drugs, e.g. neomycin, cholestyramine
Intestinal lymphangiectasia	**Anatomical defects**
Whipple's disease	Jejunal diverticulosis
Crohn's disease	Gastrocolic fistula
Impaired digestion	**Motility defects**
Chronic pancreatitis*	Scleroderma
Previous gastric and small intestinal surgery*	Diabetes mellitus
Carcinoma of the pancreas*	
Cystic fibrosis	
Enzymic defects, e.g. lipase deficiency	

**More common causes*

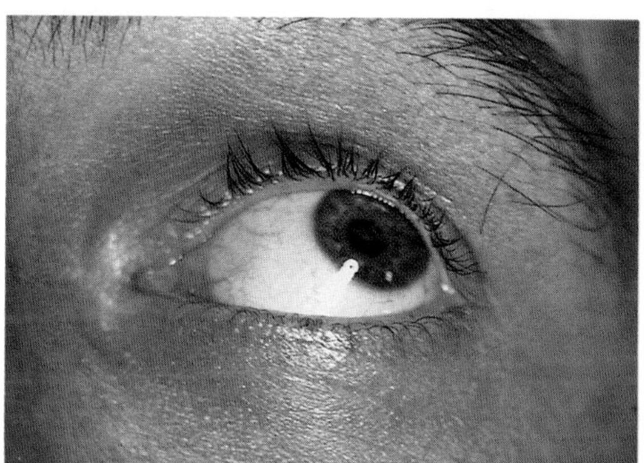

Fig. 108 Yellowing of sclera (icterus) in jaundice.

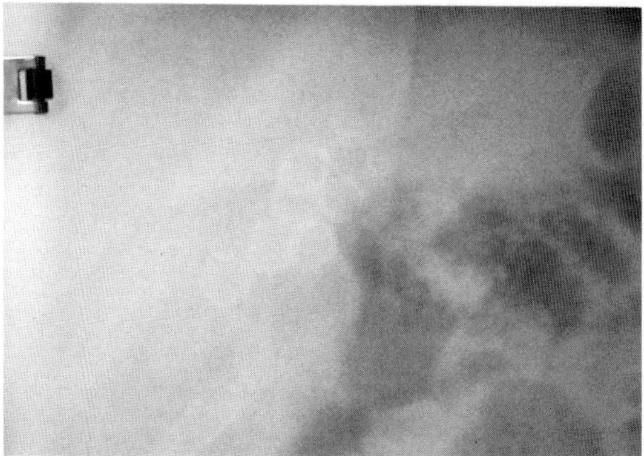

Fig. 109 Radio-opaque gallstones on abdominal radiograph.

Acute hepatitis

Aetiology

Table 12.

Clinical features

Subclinical; or anorexia, nausea, vomiting, fever, abdominal pain, jaundice (Table 13), pale stools, dark urine, pruritus.

Investigations

- Serum bilirubin, liver enzymes, viral studies.
- Occasionally biopsy, ultrasound.

Management

Rest, low protein diet, ± antivirals.

Chronic liver disease

Aetiology

Hepatitis B virus (HBV) is the main worldwide cause, but hepatitis C virus (HCV) is increasingly a cause of cirrhosis. Other non-infective causes include autoimmune disease and alcohol.

Pathology

Cirrhosis: extensive fibrosis and regeneration in nodules. Increased portal pressure produces varices (e.g. oesophageal).

Chronic active hepatitis: aggressive autoimmune disease with periportal lymphocyte infiltrate and 'piecemeal' necrosis.

Chronic persistent hepatitis: non-aggressive, little hepatic necrosis or fibrosis.

Clinical features

Sometimes asymptomatic. Features include jaundice, telangiectasia, spider naevi (Fig. 110), 'paper money' skin, purpura, pigmentation, pruritus, xanthelasma, hair loss, leuconychia, gynaecomastia. There may also be finger clubbing, Dupuytren's contracture (Fig. 111), ascites (Fig. 112, p. 84), hepatosplenomegaly, caput medusae, testicular atrophy, palmar erythema, ankle oedema, osteoporosis, muscle wasting, hepatic encephalopathy and pancytopenia and bleeding tendency.

Investigations

Similar to acute disease.

Management

When liver failure is evident:

- maintain i.v. fluid
- reduce dietary protein
- antibiotic—to clean gut of bacteria
- correct bleeding tendency.

Table 12 **Causes of acquired hepatic dysfunction**

Infections
Viral: Hepatitis viruses A, B, C, D, E, F, G, HSV, EBV, CMV, yellow fever
Bacterial: Coxiella burnetti, leptospirosis, TB, Gram-negative (ascending cholangitis)
Protozoal: Toxoplasmosis

Drugs
Almost any drug. Common ones are:
- paracetamol
- halothane

Poisons
Carbon tetrachloride
Alcohol

Trauma

Autoimmune disease
Chronic active hepatitis
Primary biliary cirrhosis

Malignancy
Hepatocellular carcinoma
Metastasis, e.g. colon, stomach, breast, bronchus

Table 13 **Causes of jaundice (icterus)**

Prehepatic
Haemolytic anaemias

Hepatic
Hepatitis (usually acute)
Cirrhosis (mild jaundice)
Congenital disease:
- Gilbert's syndrome
- Crigler–Najjar syndrome
- Dubin–Johnson syndrome
- Rotor syndrome

Post-hepatic (obstructive)
Intrahepatic
Viral hepatitis
Drugs
Alcoholic hepatitis
Cirrhosis
Pregnancy
Congenital disease
Idiopathic

Extrahepatic
Bile duct stones
Carcinoma of head of pancreas, ampulla or bile duct
Biliary stricture
Pseudocyst
Sclerosing cholangitis (autoimmune)

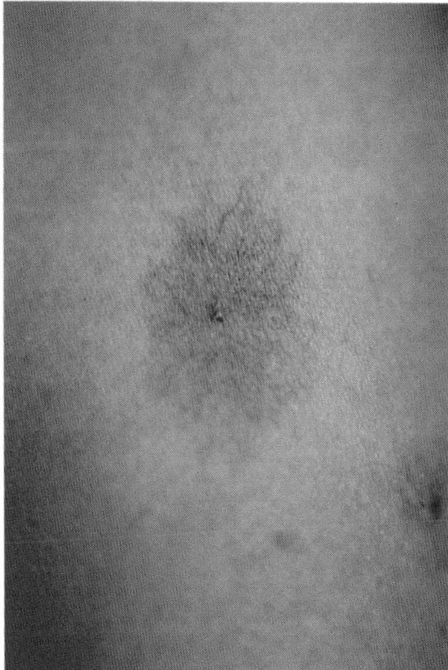

Fig. 110 A spider naevus: note the central arteriole.

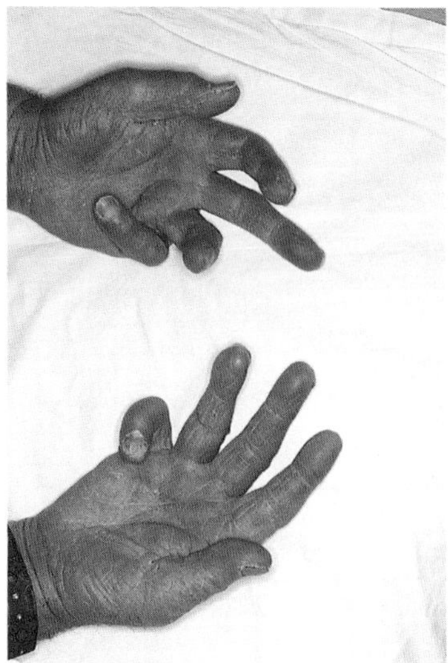

Fig. 111 Dupuytren's contractures in alcoholic cirrhosis (affects third and fourth fingers usually).

Acute pancreatitis

Aetiology

Gallstones, alcohol, viral infection (Coxsackie viruses, mumps), ischaemia, tumours, hypercalcaemia, trauma, hyperlipidaemia, drugs.

Pathology

Gallstones may block the ducts; hence proteolytic enzymes autodigest the pancreas.

Clinical features and investigations

Epigastric pain, nausea, vomiting, shock, abdominal tenderness and guarding, and ecchymoses (e.g. in umbilical area 'Cullen's sign' and on flanks 'Grey Turner's sign' (Fig. 113)). Investigations include serum amylase (raised), ultrasound, MRI or CT.

Management

Analgesia, manage shock or peritonitis, nasogastric tube, i.v. feeding, correct electrolyte disturbances.

Chronic pancreatitis

Aetiology

Alcohol, idiopathic.

Pathology

Protein plugs in ducts cause acinar atrophy and fibrosis, and calcify.

Clinical features and investigations

Epigastric pain, anorexia, weight loss, steatorrhoea, diabetes. Investigate as for acute pancreatitis, plus plain radiograph and ERCP (endoscopy).

Management

Stop alcohol intake, give analgesia, dilate obstructed ducts by endoscopy/surgery, pancreatic enzyme supplements, diabetic control.

Pancreatic cancer

Aetiology

Alcohol or tobacco.

Pathology

Adenocarcinoma—over 60% in head of pancreas (Fig. 115, p. 86). Spreads to lymph nodes and liver.

Clinical features and investigations

Jaundice; later pain, anorexia, weight loss, diabetes and other associated symptoms and signs (Fig. 114). CT/MRI is usually diagnostic.

Management

Drainage procedure and possibly surgical excision. The prognosis is very poor—2% 5-year survival.

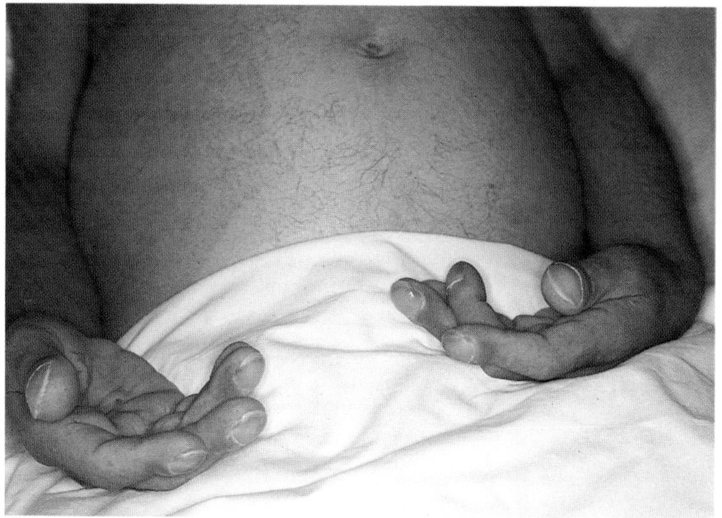

Fig. 112 Ascites and gross finger clubbing in chronic liver failure.

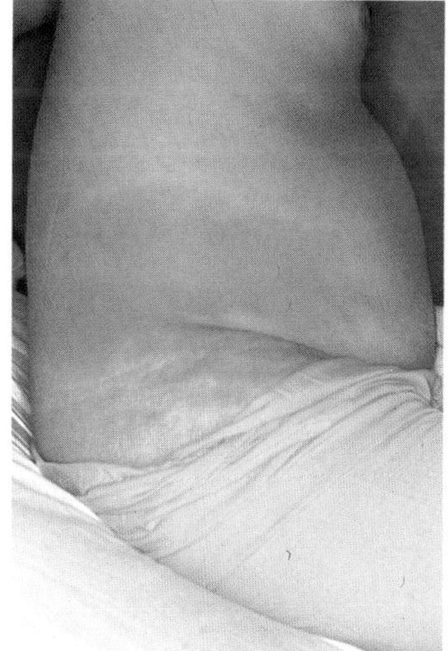

Fig. 113 Grey Turner's sign in acute pancreatitis.

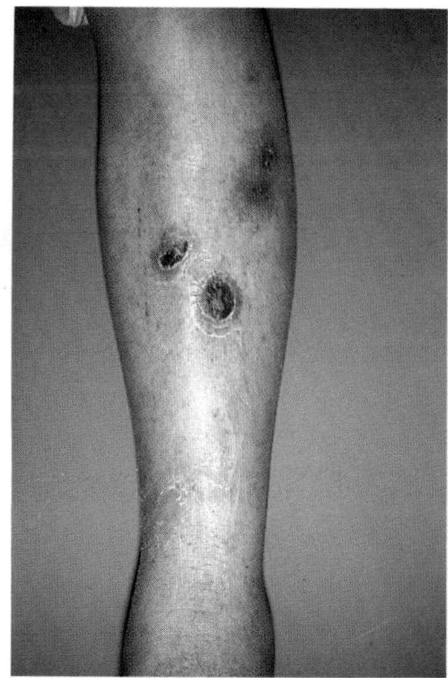

Fig. 114 Thrombophlebitis in pancreatic carcinoma.

Crohn's disease

Pathology

Aetiology unknown. Inflammation of the complete thickness of the gut lining occurs with ulcers, scarring and possibly adherence and fistula formation.

Clinical features

Crohn's disease affects mostly the terminal ileum. Pain (can mimic appendicitis), diarrhoea, weight loss, anorexia, nausea, malaise and other features (Fig. 116). Various extra-gastrointestinal features (Fig. 117) include mouth ulcers and facial swelling.

Investigations

- Blood—anaemia (various), ESR (raised).
- Barium studies (Fig. 118, p. 88), colonoscopy and biopsy.
- Stool cultures to exclude organisms (e.g. giardiasis).

Management

- Haematinic replacement.
- Salazopyrine alone; or with either (or both) systemic corticosteroids and azathioprine.
- Occasionally surgery.

Ulcerative colitis

Pathology

Extensive mucosal ulceration and polyp formation. The entire colon, *particularly* the rectum, can be affected.

Clinical features

Similar to Crohn's disease but without fistulae or abscesses. The condition is characterized by typical mucus-containing (slime-like) often bloody diarrhoea. There are also extragastrointestinal features.

Investigations/ management

Similar to Crohn's disease but colectomy can be curative.

Complications

Liability to colonic carcinoma.

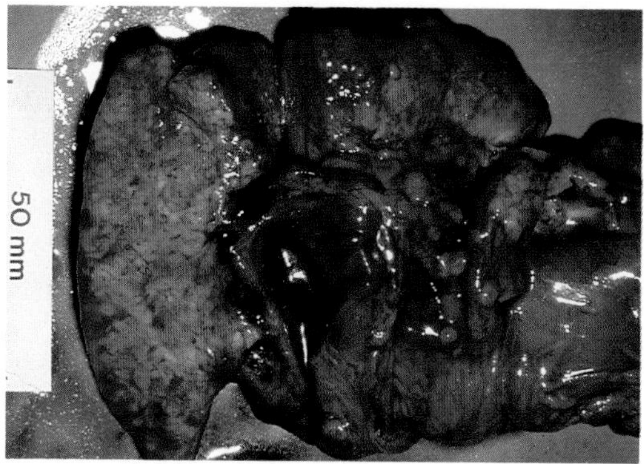

Fig. 115 Pancreatic carcinoma in postmortem specimen.

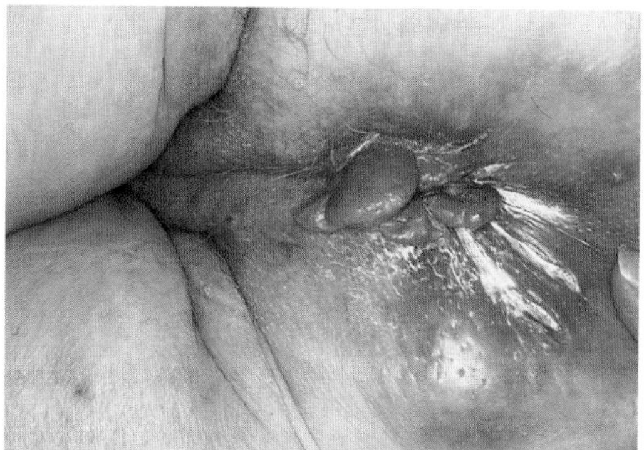

Fig. 116 Anal skin tags, fistula, perianal discoloration in Crohn's disease.

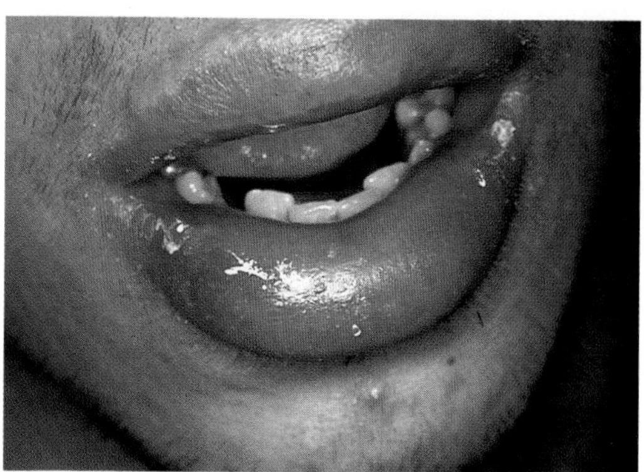

Fig. 117 Labial swelling in Crohn's disease.

Colorectal carcinoma

Aetiology — High animal fat, low fibre diet and long-standing ulcerative colitis.

Pathology — Majority are adenocarcinomas (Fig. 119).

Clinical features

- Bleeding from rectum.
- Constipation or diarrhoea.
- Tenesmus (sensation of incomplete evacuation).
- Anorexia, weight loss, anaemia.

Investigations — Proctosigmoidoscopy, colonoscopy, barium studies (Fig. 120), biopsy, liver ultrasound, full blood picture, faecal occult bloods, CT/MRI.

Management — Surgery, occasionally with chemotherapy.

Irritable bowel syndrome

Aetiology — Symptoms of lower gut dysfunction, in the absence of demonstrable organic pathology.

Clinical features

- Pain in iliac fossa, with some relief on defaecation.
- Frequent urge to defaecate.
- Stools loose, or pellet-like.
- Many have a 'morning rush', defaecating several times.

Management — High fibre diet, antispasmodics, antidiarrhoeals.

Intussusception

Aetiology — Idiopathic, hyperplasia of mesenteric lymph nodes, carcinoma or Meckel's diverticulum.

Pathology — Invagination of bowel into adjacent bowel leads to necrosis or obstruction.

Clinical features

- Pain in iliac fossa, with some relief on defaecation.
- Bleeding from rectum, 'red-currant jelly' stools.
- Sausage-shaped abdominal mass.

Investigation — Barium enema in atypical presentations.

Management — Correction by barium enema or surgery.

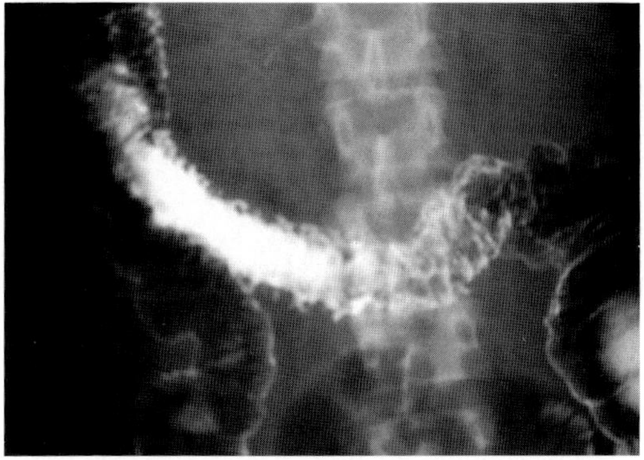

Fig. 118 Barium studies: Crohn's disease.

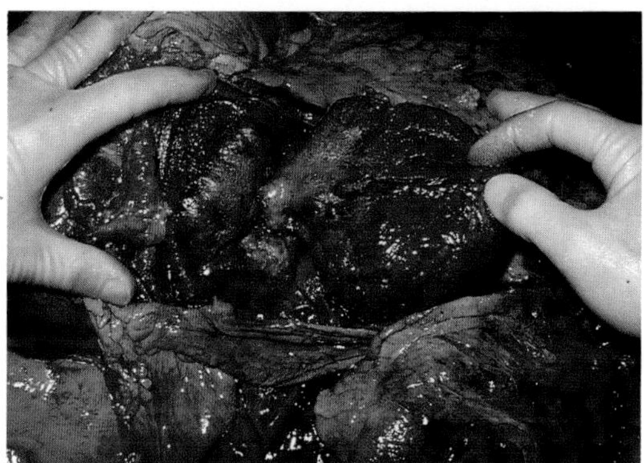

Fig. 119 Colonic carcinoma: operative specimen.

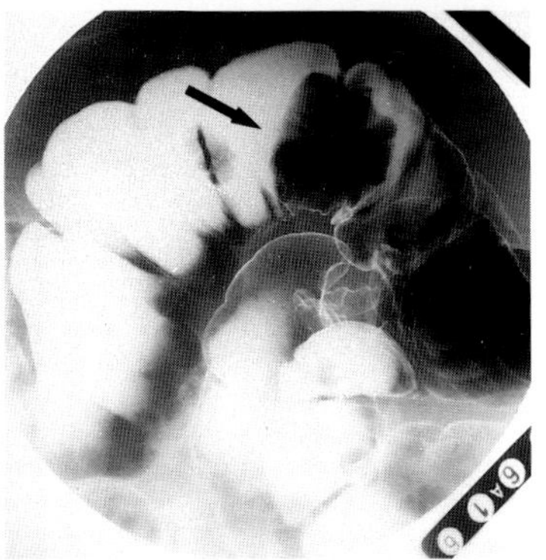

Fig. 120 Barium enema showing large colonic carcinoma.

Diverticular disease

Pathology — Mucosal outpouches of the sigmoid colon.

Clinical features — Often symptomless. In acute diverticulitis there is pain in the left iliac fossa, pyrexia, constipation and tenderness, guarding and rigidity.

Investigations — Barium enema or more rarely colonoscopy.

Management — High fibre diet, possibly antispasmodics.

Volvulus

Aetiology — Congenital, tumours, constipation and adhesions secondary to surgery.

Pathology — Twisting of mesentery occludes the blood supply and intestine.

Clinical features — Sudden pain, gross dilatation of abdomen (Fig. 121).

Investigations — Plain radiographs.

Management — Sigmoidoscopic decompression may be curative, otherwise laparotomy is necessary.

Appendicitis

Pathology — Obstruction of lumen by faecoliths; or lymphoid hyperplasia causing ischaemia. There is eventual abscess formation and peritonitis.

Clinical features — Central pain that moves to right iliac fossa (McBurney's point, Fig. 122); nausea, vomiting and pyrexia.

Investigations — Of little value, although ultrasound can be used to localize a mass.

Management — Appendicectomy.

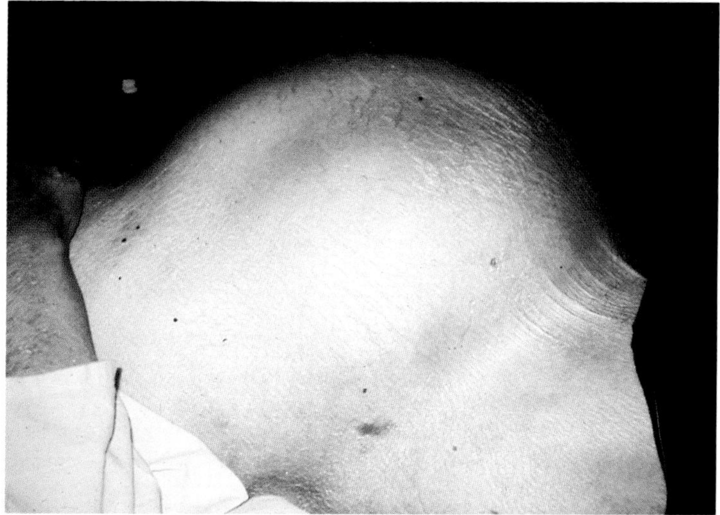

Fig. 121 Gross example of abdominal swelling due to volvulus.

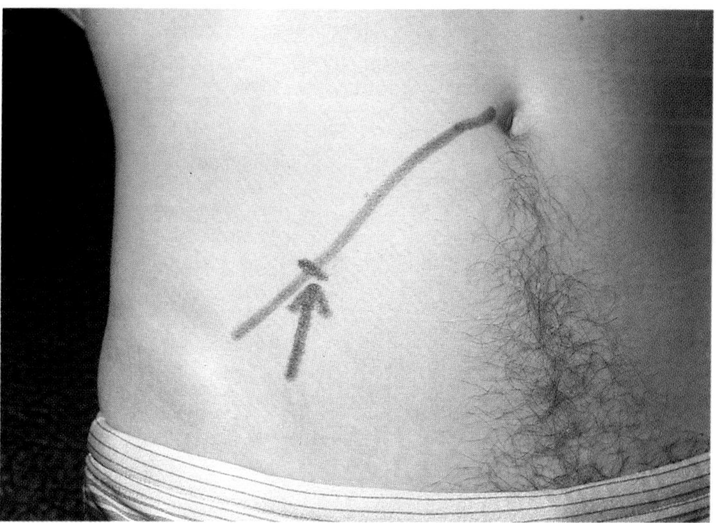

Fig. 122 McBurney's point: common site of pain of appendicitis.

9 / Breast disease

Breast cancer

Aetiology

Unknown. There is a genetic predisposition in some, other risk factors include malignancy in the opposite breast, smoking, non-parity, early menarche and late menopause, chest radiotherapy.

Pathology

Usually ductal adenocarcinomas (Fig. 123).

Clinical features

Pain; lump; ulcer; nipple inversion, discharge or bleeding; axillary or supraclavicular lymphadenopathy (Fig. 124); or lymph obstruction. Metastases may cause weight loss, anaemia, jaundice or pathological fracture.

Investigations

- Fine needle aspiration or excisional biopsy (i.e. lumpectomy).
- Mammography.
- Plain chest radiograph and liver ultrasound.
- Bone scan if widespread bone metastases likely.

Management

- Surgery plus radiotherapy (Fig. 125).
- Anti-oestrogen (tamoxifen) therapy in hormone-dependent cases.

Prognosis

Variable. Single lesions without nodal involvement have a greater than 90% 5-year survival. Nodal involvement decreases 5-year survival to under 50%. Metastatic disease indicates poor 5-year survival. Even patients with supposed local disease can eventually develop metastases up to 20 years after successful local clearance.

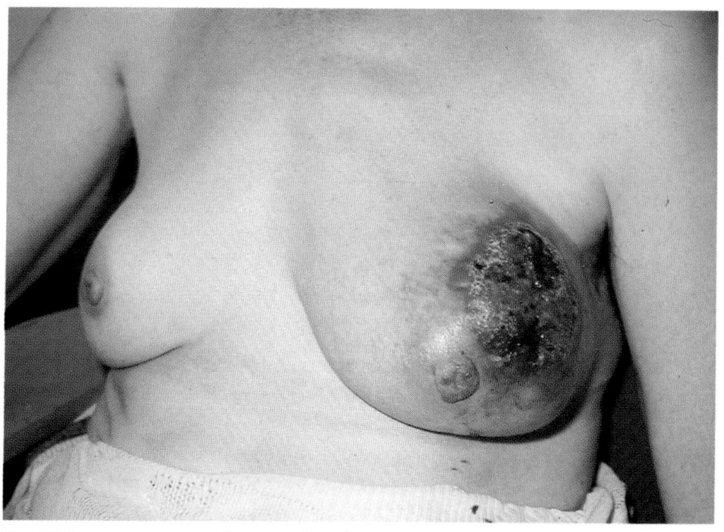

Fig. 123 Breast cancer: usually a ductal carcinoma.

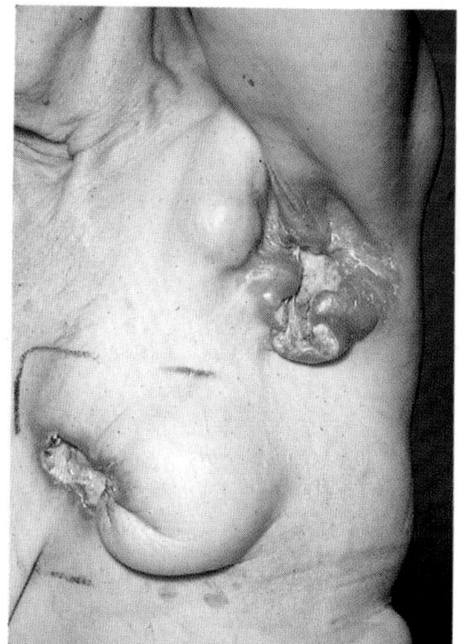

Fig. 124 Breast cancer with involvement of axillary nodes.

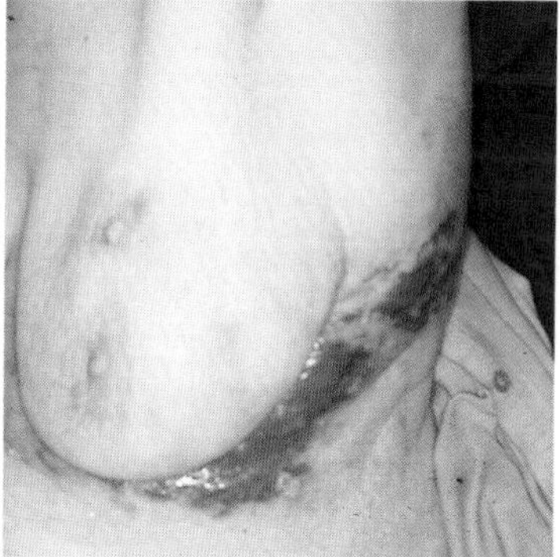

Fig. 125 Shingles secondary to radiotherapy for carcinoma of breast.

10 / Endocrine disease

Diabetes mellitus

Epidemiology

- *Type I (insulin-dependent):* onset in the young.
- *Type II:* onset in middle to late life.

Aetiology

Viral and/or autoimmune basis has been suggested. Some diseases/drugs predispose.

Pathology

Insufficient insulin causes low intracellular glucose (despite hyperglycaemia). Fats are therefore metabolized to ketones, with acidosis.

Clinical features

Initially symptomless. Polyuria, polydipsia and weight loss develop with, later, coma, dehydration, tachypnoea and ketones on breath. Patients may present with complications of the disease or may be identified following routine urinalysis.

Complications

Liability to coma, atherosclerosis, ocular disease (Fig. 126), peripheral vascular disease, renal disease, neuropathies and infections.

Diagnosis

- Glycosuria.
- Raised random or fasting blood glucose, glycosylated haemoglobin, or serum fructosamine.
- Abnormal response in glucose tolerance test—prolonged elevated serum glucose.

Management

- *Type I:* diet (e.g. restrict sugars and excess fat) and insulin injections.
- *Type II:* diet and oral hypoglycaemics (usually).

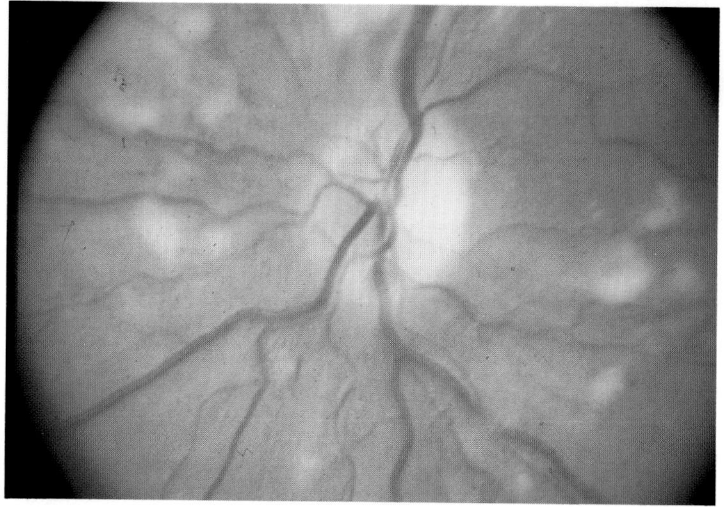

Fig. 126 Soft retinal exudates in diabetes mellitus.

Growth hormone excess

Pathology

Acidophil adenoma of anterior pituitary.

Clinical features

Acromegaly—prominent supraorbital ridges, visual field defects, headaches, prognathism, enlarged tongue, spaced teeth, goitre, broad nose (Fig. 127), hypertension, cardiac failure, enlarged fingers (Fig. 129) and toes, diabetes mellitus, carpal tunnel syndrome, proximal myopathy.

Investigations

- CT or MRI of pituitary (Fig. 128).
- Visual field testing—loss of temporal fields (bitemporal hemianopia or 'tunnel vision').
- Growth hormone levels (raised).

Management

Radiotherapy or surgery of pituitary adenoma.

Growth hormone deficiency

Aetiology

Tumour, meningitis, trauma, or post-partum ischaemia (Sheehan syndrome).

Clinical features

In children, failure to grow. In adults, secondary amenorrhoea and adrenal cortex failure.

Investigations

- Growth hormone levels (low).
- Insulin exposure.
- Radiological examination of hands.

Management

Replacement therapy.

Diabetes insipidus

Aetiology

Inadequate antidiuretic hormone (ADH) due to trauma, tumour, infection or infiltrations (e.g. sarcoidosis).

Clinical features

Polydipsia, polyuria, nocturia.

Investigations

Reduced plasma osmolality and sodium. Reduced concentration of urine despite fluid restriction, yet restored with ADH.

Management

Synthetic ADH.

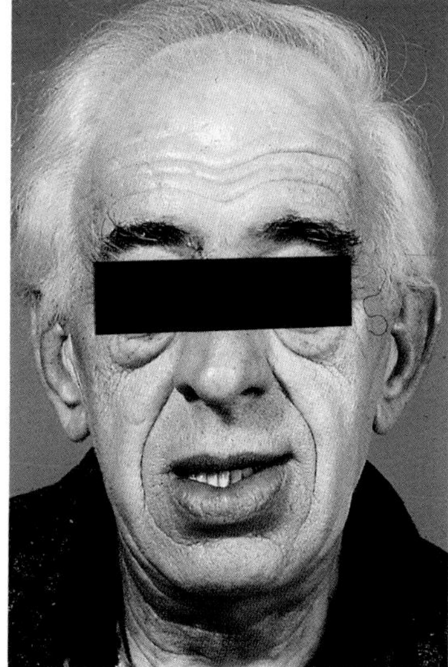

Fig. 127 Coarse features secondary to acromegaly.

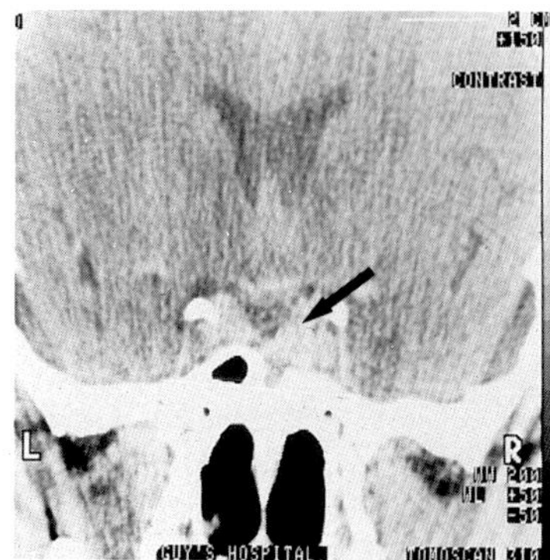

Fig. 128 Coronal CT of the pituitary fossa showing an adenoma in acromegaly.

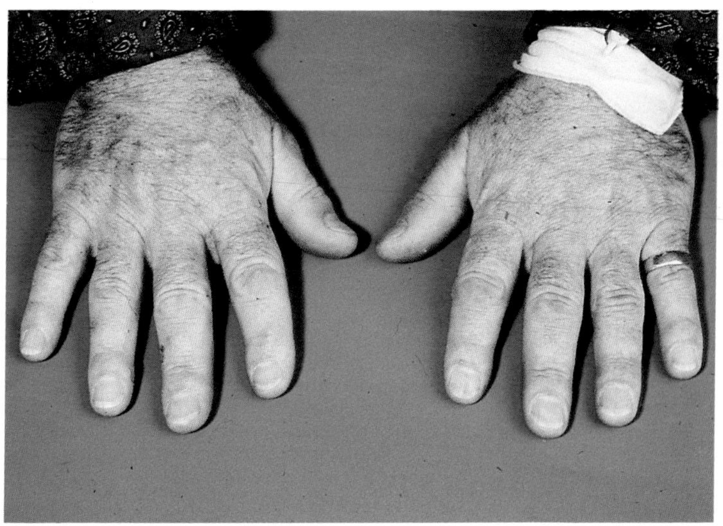

Fig. 129 Typical spade-like hands associated with acromegaly.

Hyperthyroidism

Aetiology

Graves' disease (autoimmune) (Fig. 130), adenomas, toxic goitre, acute thyroiditis, exogenous thyroxine, or thyroid-stimulating hormone (TSH)-producing tumours.

Clinical features

Table 14.

Investigations

- Raised T_3, T_4; usually decreased TSH.
- Autoantibodies.
- Radioactive iodine scan.

Management

Surgery, carbimazole or radioiodine.

Hypothyroidism (myxoedema)

Aetiology

Agenesis, or hypoplasia, autoimmune disease, infection, surgery, irradiation, antithyroid drugs, iodine deficiency.

Clinical features

Table 14, Figs 131 & 132.

Investigations

- Reduced T_3, T_4; elevated TSH.
- Antibodies to thyroid microsomes or thyroglobulin.

Management

Thyroxine.

Goitre

Definition

Thyroid enlargement.

Aetiology

Physiological: e.g. puberty, pregnancy.

Pathological: iodine deficiency, drugs, autoimmune disease.

Clinical features

Gland enlarged, and tender in acute thyroiditis. Goitre in chronic thyroiditis and neoplasia can compress trachea or oesophagus. A retrosternal goitre can produce venous dilatation on the chest (Fig. 133, p. 100).

Investigations

- T_3, T_4 (reduced); TSH (variable); iodine (variable).
- Thyroid scan; ultrasound.
- Biopsy.

Treatment

Low dose thyroxine (to suppress endogenous TSH), or surgery.

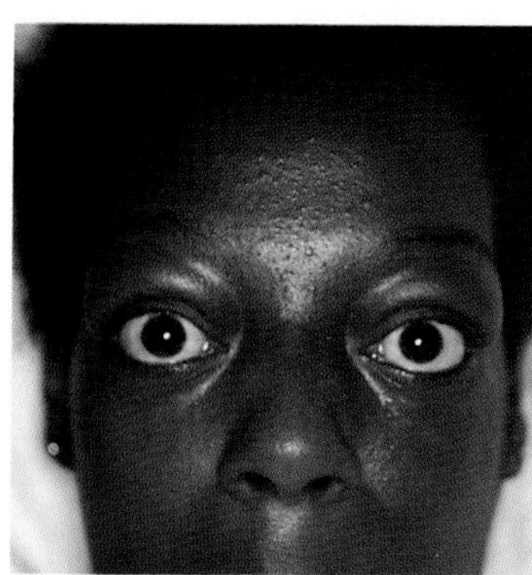

Fig. 130 Exophthalmos in Graves' disease.

Table 14 **Clinical features of hypo- and hyperthyroidism**

Hypothyroidism	Hyperthyroidism
Cold intolerance	Heat intolerance
Decreased sweating	Excess sweating
Dry cold skin	Warm moist skin
Loss of hair	Pretibial myxoedema
Periorbital myxoedema (Figs 131 & 132)	Increased appetite
Decreased appetite	Weight loss
Weight gain	Tachycardia (atrial fibrillation)
Bradycardia	Heart failure
Angina	Tremor
Hoarseness	Diarrhoea
Slow reactions/reflexes	Irritability
Constipation	Psychosis
Slow cerebration	Amenorrhoea
Poor memory	
Psychosis	

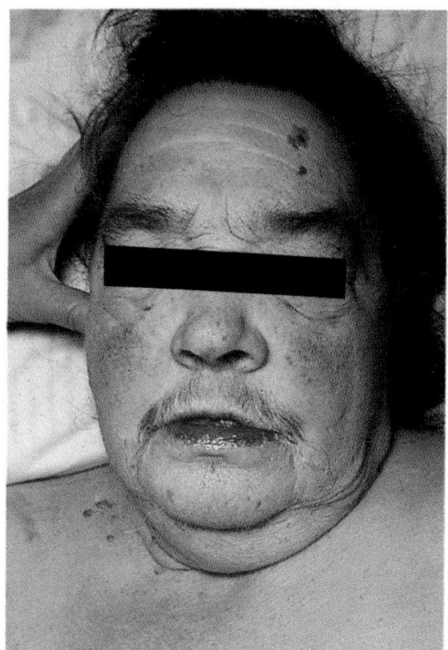

Fig. 131 Myxoedema (hypothyroidism).

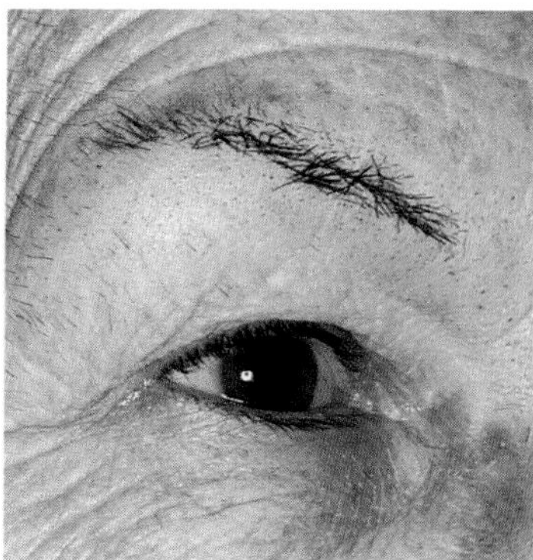

Fig. 132 Hair loss of myxoedema.

Hyperadrenocorticism

Aetiology

Pituitary tumour (Cushing syndrome), ectopic adrenocorticotrophic hormone (ACTH) production from various tumours or adrenal tumours.

Clinical features and investigations

Increased weight, hypertension, redistribution of fat (e.g. moonface, Fig. 134, buffalo hump, Fig. 135), acne, striae, poor healing, osteoporosis, and myopathy, diabetogenic status, depression and infection susceptibility (same can happen in corticosteroid therapy).

Management

Manage underlying cause.

Mineralocorticoid excess

Aetiology

Adrenal adenoma (Conn syndrome) or hyperplasia.

Clinical features

Hypertension, increased serum Na, reduced K.

Management

Remove adenoma. Treat with aldosterone antagonist (spironolactone) in adrenal hyperplasia.

Hypoadrenocorticism (Addison's disease)

Aetiology

Adrenal hypoplasia, autoimmunity, infection, tumour, enzyme defects.

Clinical features and investigations

Anorexia, nausea, abdominal pain, weakness, hyperpigmentation (Fig. 136), weight loss, hypotension, impotence or amenorrhoea.

- Serum sodium (reduced); potassium (raised).
- Low plasma cortisol and failed elevation after ACTH (Synacthen test).

Management

Corticosteroids.

Phaeochromocytoma

Pathology

Benign tumour of adrenal medulla.

Clinical features

Panic, palpitations, tremor, headache, flushing, nausea, vomiting, weight loss, diarrhoea or constipation. Sometimes multiple endocrinopathies.

Management

Remove tumour.

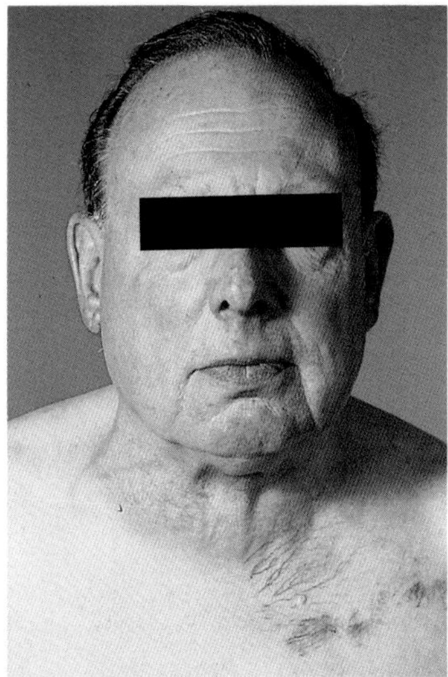

Fig. 133 Retrosternal goitre causing venous dilatation on left side of chest.

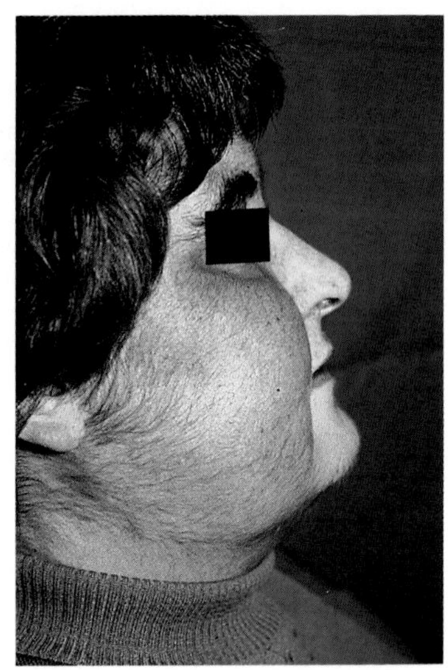

Fig. 134 Hirsutism and moonface in Cushing syndrome.

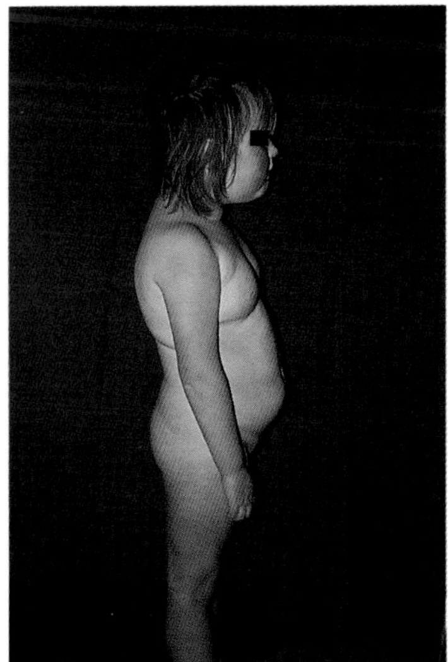

Fig. 135 Truncal obesity, gynaecomastia, buffalo hump and acne in Cushing syndrome.

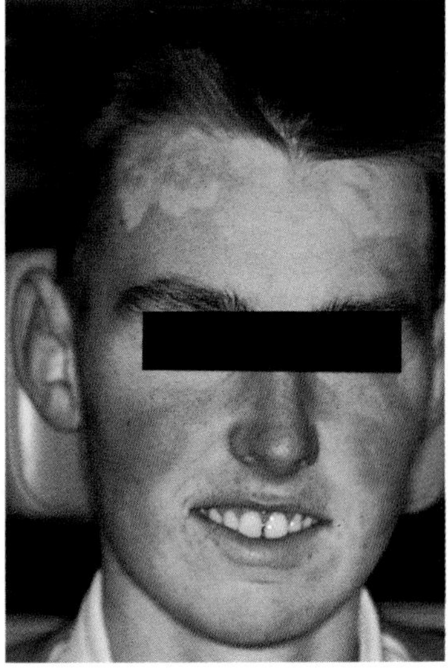

Fig. 136 Addisonian pigmentation and vitiligo.

Hyperparathyroidism

Aetiology

Primary hyperparathyroidism: parathyroid adenoma.

Secondary hyperparathyroidism: malabsorption, vitamin D deficiency or chronic renal disease.

Clinical features/ Investigations

Table 15. Serum calcium, phosphate and alkaline phosphatase may delineate types—hypophosphataemia in primary disease; serum parathyroid hormone levels (raised); radiographs for renal calculi and subperiosteal erosions of fingers (Fig. 137).

Management

- *Primary:* surgery.
- *Secondary:* correct cause, then calcium and vitamin D supplements.

Hypoparathyroidism

Aetiology

Agenesis, post-surgery, autoimmune disease.

Clinical features/ Investigations

Table 15. Serum calcium (reduced), phosphate (raised), parathyroid hormone (reduced); parathyroid antibodies.

Management

Calcium and vitamin D supplements.

Vitamin D deficiency

Aetiology

Inadequate exposure to sun combined with low calcium or calcium-blocking diet (chupattis); renal or liver disease.

Clinical features

Childhood—rickets: reduced stature, bone pain, enlarged metaphyses, hyperplasia of costochondral cartilages, delayed closure of fontanelles, soft skull bones and bending of long bones (Figs 138 & 139).

Adulthood—osteomalacia: bone and muscle pain, increased liability to fracture.

Investigations

Serum calcium and phosphate (reduced) and alkaline phosphatase (elevated); radiographs show loss of mineralization and pseudofractures—Looser's zones.

Management

Vitamin D supplements.

Table 15 **Clinical features of hyper- and hypoparathyroidism**

Hyperparathyroidism	Hypoparathyroidism
Renal stones	Tetany*
Nephrocalcinosis	Epilepsy
Bone resorption	Candidosis[†]
Peptic ulcer pain	Cataracts[†]
Psychiatric disorders	Psychiatric disorders
Polyuria	
Constipation	
Hypertension	
Weakness	
Acute pancreatitis	

**Chvostek's sign: tapping of the facial nerve induces facial twitching; Trousseau's sign: inflation of the sphygmomanometer about forearm above diastolic pressure for 3 min induces spasm of the fingers and wrist (the obstetrician's hand).*
[†]Only in some types of congenital hypoparathyroidism

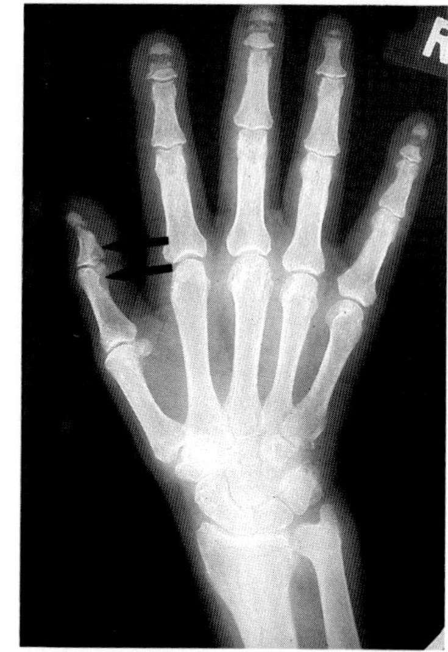

Fig. 137 Subperiosteal erosions in hyperparathyroidism.

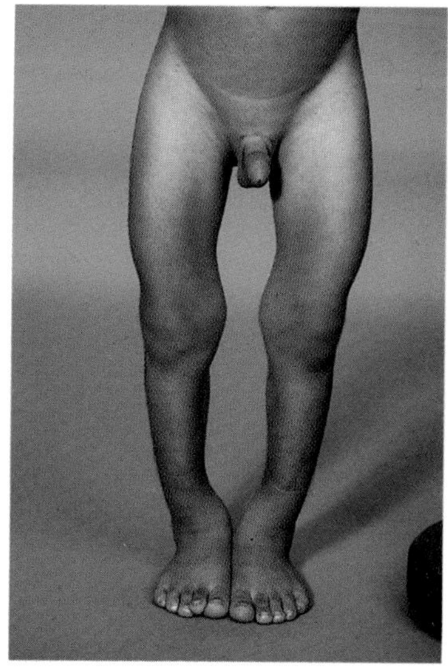

Fig. 138 Genu varus (bow legs) due to rickets.

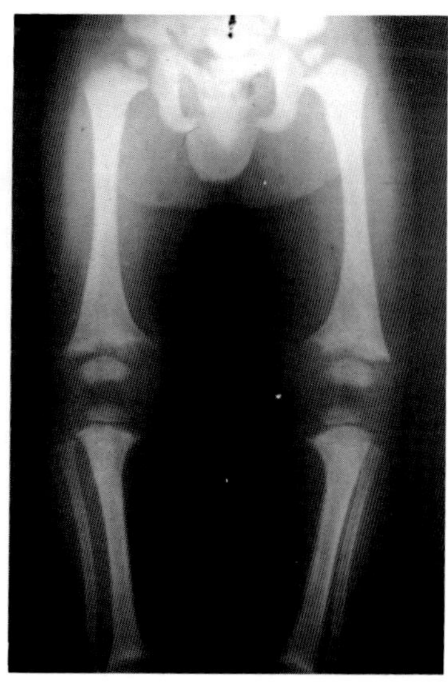

Fig. 139 Rickets.

11 / Genitourinary disease

Urinary tract infection

Aetiology Infection from sexual intercourse ('honeymoon cystitis'), poor hygiene, catheterization.

Clinical features Dysuria, frequency, nocturia, haematuria (Table 16), pyuria and smelly urine; suprapubic pain.

Investigations Microscopy and culture of midstream sample of urine (MSSU).

Management Fluids; antibiotics.

Pyelonephritis

Aetiology Reflux of infected urine up the ureter can cause secondary infection of renal pelvis and possibly parenchyma (pyelonephritis).

Clinical features Pyrexia, loin pain. There may be hypertension in later life if severe disease has caused gross renal scarring.

Investigations

- MSSU.
- Intravenous urography (IVU).

Management Eradicate infection; treat any renal failure.

Nephrotic syndrome

Aetiology Glomerulonephritis, systemic lupus erythematosus, diabetes, renal vein thrombosis, syphilis.

Clinical features Profound oedema affecting face, arms and genitalia, and ascites.

Investigations

- Proteinuria (24 h urinary protein).
- Serum albumin concentration (reduced).
- Renal biopsy may be needed.

Management Systemic corticosteroids or cyclophosphamide.

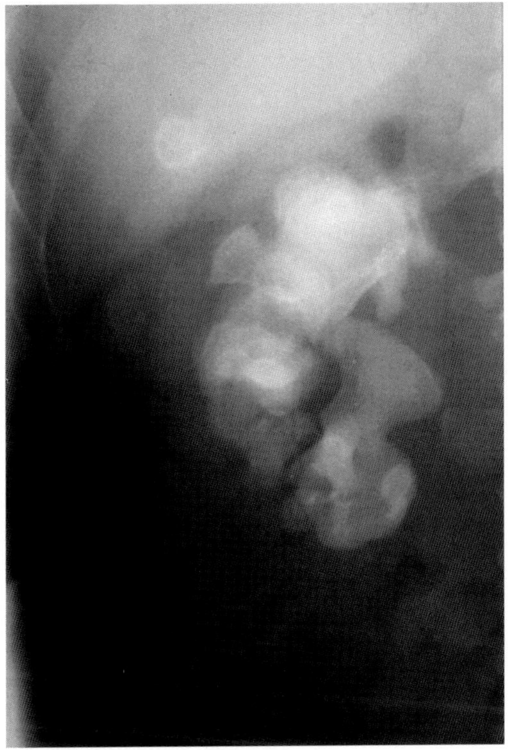

Fig. 140 Staghorn renal calculus.

Table 16 **Causes of haematuria (blood in urine)**

Kidney	**Bladder and urethra**
Trauma	Calculi
Calculi	Neoplasms
Cysts	Trauma
Glomerulonephritis	Infection
Carcinoma	
Idiopathic	**Other**
	Bleeding tendency
Ureter	Drugs
Calculi	
Neoplasms	

Acute renal failure (ARF: acute uraemia)

Definition — Urine output of less than 400 ml/24 h.

Aetiology — *Prerenal uraemia:* poor kidney perfusion due to hypotension/hypovolaemia, or cardiac failure.

Renal uraemia: glomerular or medullary disease.

Post-renal uraemia: urinary obstruction/infection (Fig. 140, p. 104).

Clinical features — Oliguria or anuria.

Investigations

- Serum urea, creatinine and potassium (all rising).
- Urine output (falling), creatinine clearance (reduced).
- Plain radiographs/ultrasound/intravenous urogram.

Management

- Restrict proteins and fluids.
- Correct electrolytes.

Chronic renal failure

Aetiology — As acute renal failure.

Clinical features — Anorexia, lethargy, malaise, vomiting, epistaxis, weight loss, hypertension, anaemia.

Investigations — As acute renal failure.

Management

- Low dietary protein, high fluids plus diuretic (frusemide), vitamin D supplements.
- Correct electrolyte disturbances.
- Consider dialysis (Figs 141 & 142) or renal transplant.

Benign prostatic enlargement

Pathology — Hypertrophy of prostate—aetiology unknown.

Clinical features — Difficulty in initiating urination (hesitancy), poor stream.

Management — Acute urinary retention requires catherization. Alpha-reductase inhibitors may help. Hypertrophy usually necessitates transurethral resection of prostate (TURP).

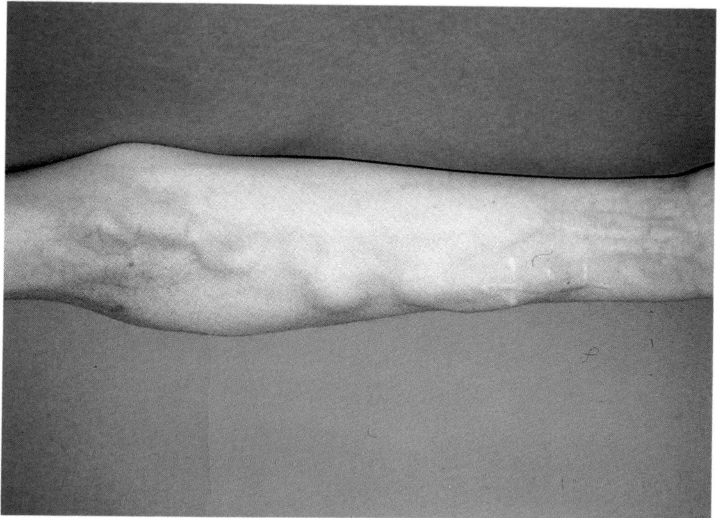

Fig. 141 Arteriovenous shunt to facilitate haemodialysis.

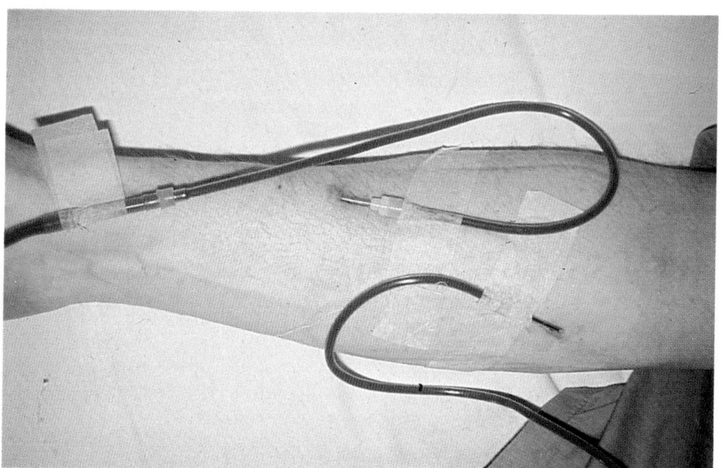

Fig. 142 Haemodialysis in progress.

Prostatic carcinoma

Aetiology May have hormonal (androgen) basis.

Pathology Adenocarcinoma.

Clinical features Poor urinary stream, hesitancy, obstruction; hard mass on rectal examination; metastasizes mainly to bone.

Investigations

- Biopsy via needle aspiration or transurethral resection.
- Raised prostate-specific antigen (PSA).
- Ultrasound/CT—bone metastases, typically osteosclerotic, in pelvis and upper femur.

Management Prostatectomy and/or orchidectomy, radiotherapy, chemotherapy (including gonadorelins or anti-androgens).

Bladder carcinoma

Aetiology Naphthylamine; benzidine; drugs; chronic inflammation (e.g. schistosomiasis).

Pathology Transitional cell carcinoma.

Clinical features Commonly painless haematuria. Obstruction by clot may cause pain.

Investigations

- Intravenous urography (Fig. 143).
- Cystoscopy for biopsy (with or without CT).

Management Cystodiathermy with or without local cytotoxics, or cystectomy.

Testicular torsion

Aetiology Idiopathic but predisposing factors include ectopic testis, horizontal ('clapper bell') testis, well-developed spiral cremaster muscle.

Clinical features Sudden onset of lower abdominal and testicular pain, usually in a young adult. The testis is swollen, tender, elevated and red.

Management Emergency surgical correction; also fix contralateral testis to prevent torsion.

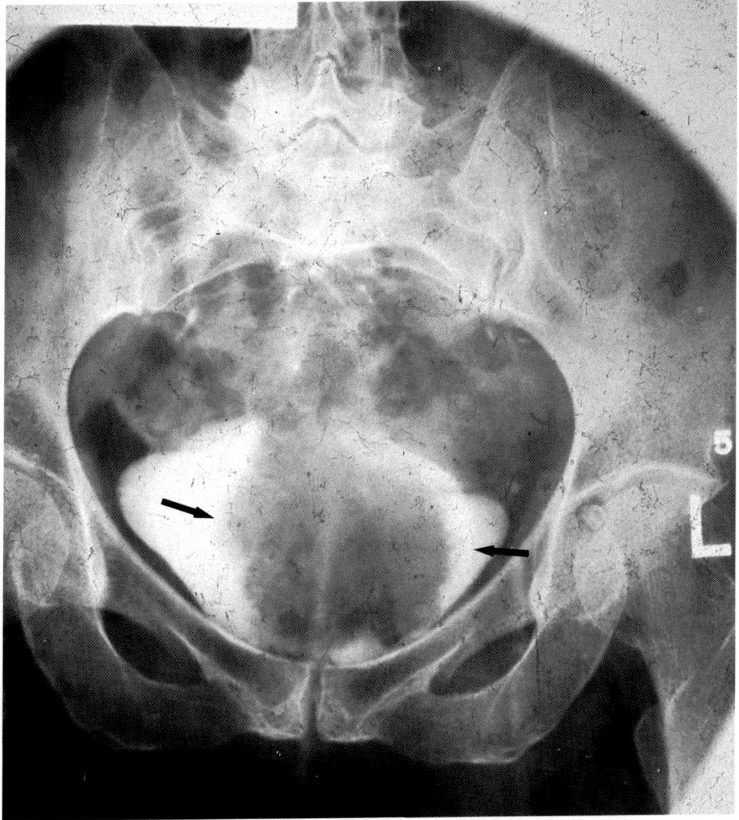

Fig. 143 Large bladder carcinoma: delineated by intravenous urography (IVU).

Scrotal and groin swellings

Inguinal hernia

Herniation of peritoneum, omentum and sometimes gut into the inguinal canal (Fig. 144). Treatment is by herniorrhaphy (usually).

Femoral hernia

Herniation of peritoneum, omentum and sometimes gut into the femoral canal. A femoral hernia is prone to strangulation and requires herniorrhaphy.

Varicocele

Dilatation of the venous plexus above the testis, like a 'can of worms'. Varicoceles account for 10% of male infertility. Surgery may be required.

Hydrocele

Fluid-filled swelling of the tunica vaginalis of the testis. It can be idiopathic, congenital, traumatic, or neoplastic in origin. Surgery may be required.

Ectopic testis

An *undescended* testis can lie intra-abdominally, within the inguinal canal or high within the scrotum. The affected testis is small and sterile. A *maldescended* testis descends abnormally outside the superficial inguinal ring. Both have increased risk of malignancy. Both warrant surgery.

Testicular neoplasia

Seminoma or teratoma which presents with swelling, tenderness, or para-aortic lymphadenopathy.

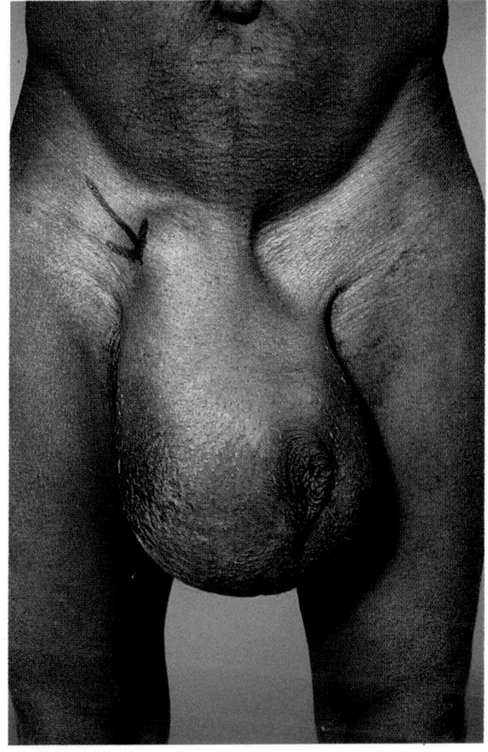

Fig. 144 Gross inguinal hernia.

12 / Neurological disease

Cerebrovascular accident (CVA: stroke)

Aetiology

Thrombosis, embolism, or haemorrhage from a cerebral artery. Hypertension, diabetes, smoking and the contraceptive pill predispose.

Pathology

Infarction of part of brain.

Clinical features

Upper motor neurone lesion—specific features depend on site (Table 17).

Investigations

- ECG, pulse and BP.
- Chest radiograph.
- Blood cultures, blood sugar, full blood picture, syphilis serology.
- CT scan, carotid Doppler.

Management

- Relieve distress.
- Nursing and physiotherapy.
- Correct any underlying cause.

Epilepsy

Aetiology

Often no cause can be identified. Identifiable causes are: trauma; tumours; infections; metabolic causes or drugs.

Clinical features

Generalized epilepsy (grand mal): loss of consciousness; tonic then clonic spasms, possibly with urinary and/or faecal incontinence; then recovery.

Petit mal: brief 'absences' of up to 10 s—usually in a child of 5–9 years.

Focal motor epilepsy: twitching of face, arm or leg.

Temporal lobe epilepsy: altered sensory awareness; stereotypic behaviour; automatism.

Myoclonic epilepsy: contractions of muscles or groups of muscles.

Infantile spasms: flexion spasms in infant. The electroencephalogram (EEG) is characteristic.

Investigations

Neurological examination with CT/MRI scan and EEG.

Management

Anticonvulsants, such as phenytoin (Fig. 145).

Table 17 **Main features of specific cerebrovascular accidents**

Location	Features
Middle cerebral artery (most common) or internal carotid artery	Contralateral hemiplegia Sensory loss of face ± dysphasia (if affecting dominant side)
Anterior cerebral artery	Contralateral lower limb weakness
Posterior cerebral artery	Contralateral visual defect (homonymous hemianopia)
Basilar artery	Ouadraplegia, coma, death
Midbrain infarct	Coma, oculomotor nerve palsy, hemi- or quadraplegia

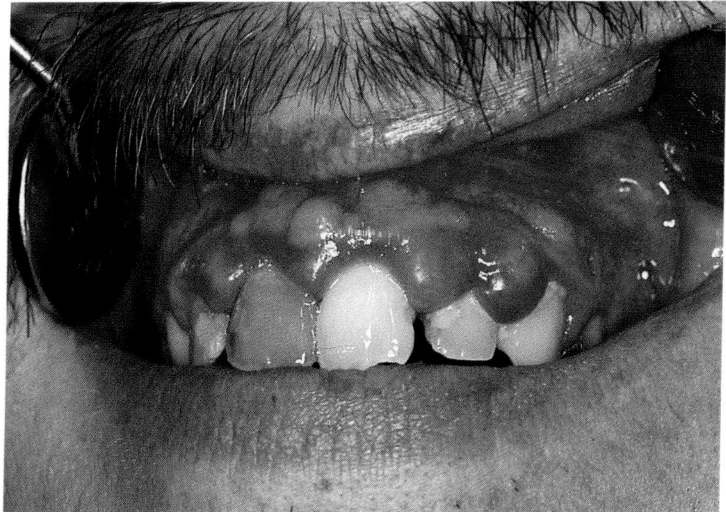

Fig. 145 Gingival hyperplasia secondary to phenytoin treatment for epilepsy. The discoloured tooth resulted from pulp necrosis following damage in a grand mal fit.

Multiple (disseminated) sclerosis

Aetiology and pathology

Unknown causes, possibly viral. Multiple plaques of demyelination in CNS—particularly the optic nerve, brain stem, periventricular sites and cerebellum.

Clinical features

Lesions are disseminated in time and place. Typically there is: optic (retrobulbar) neuritis—unilateral with rapid loss of (central) vision; isolated numbness or weakness.

Investigations

Polyclonal immunoglobulins in cerebrospinal fluid (CSF). MRI can delineate plaques (Fig. 146).

Management

Acute disease is treated with ACTH or prednisolone. Physiotherapy and nursing support are important for maintenance (Fig. 147).

Prognosis

Highly variable. Some have single episodes of reversible illness; in others the disease is relentlessly progressive.

Parkinson's disease

Aetiology and pathology

Usually idiopathic. Arteriosclerosis, chronic trauma (boxers), encephalitis lethargica and drugs (e.g. phenothiazines) are other causes. Defect in dopaminergic neurones in basal ganglia and midbrain.

Clinical features

- *Hypokinesia*—slowness in initiating and performing movements.
- *Tremor*—affecting fingers at rest ('pill rolling').
- *Rigidity*—('lead-pipe' rigidity) sometimes with superimposed tremor ('cogwheel' rigidity).

The condition manifests itself in: small writing (micrographia); expressionless (mask-like) face; impaired blink reflex; and shuffling (festinant) gait (Fig. 148). The speech is slow and quiet.

Management

L-dopa plus dopa decarboxylase inhibitor (carbidopa); dopaminergic agonist (selegiline); anticholinergics (e.g. benzhexol) relieve tremor.

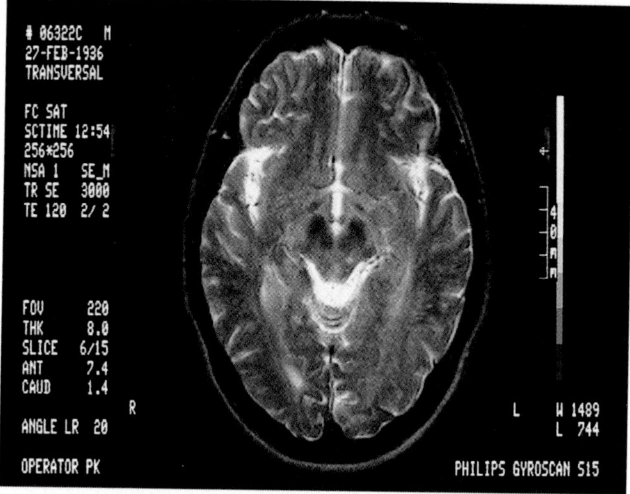

Fig. 146 MRI delineating multiple plaques of demyelination throughout the brain parenchyma in multiple sclerosis.

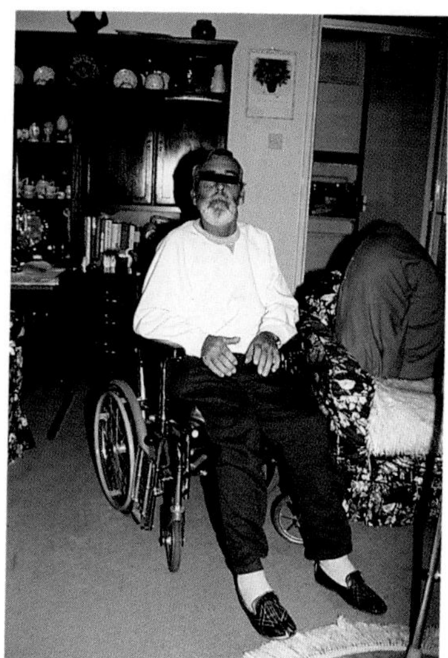

Fig. 147 Multiple sclerosis: paraplegia.

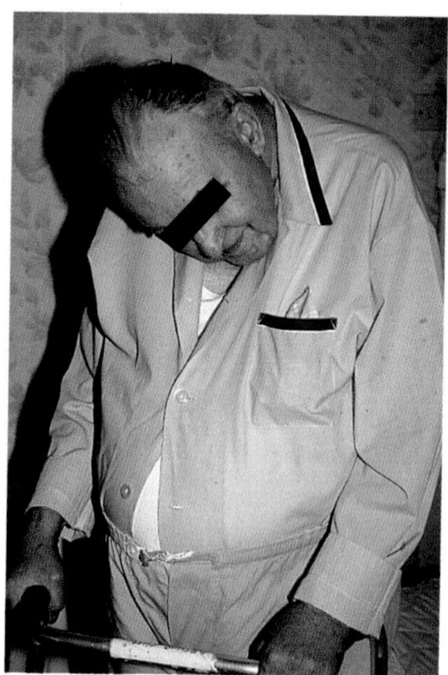

Fig. 148 Parkinson's disease.

Meningitis

Aetiology

Viruses: Most commonly, e.g. Coxsackie.

Bacteria:

- neonates—*Escherichia coli, Listeria monocytogenes*
- children—*Haemophilus influenzae* (Hib), *Neisseria meningitidis*
- middle age—*N. meningitidis, Streptococcus pneumoniae, Mycobacterium tuberculosis*
- elderly—*L. monocytogenes*

Pathology

Infection of the pia and arachnoid mater. The CSF contains organisms, and in 'bacterial meningitis' there are many neutrophils and reduced glucose in CSF.

Clinical features

- Severe persistent headache.
- Pain and stiffness of neck (Fig. 149).
- Kernig's sign—pain in hamstrings on *extending* knee when hip flexed.
- Vomiting, photophobia, fever.
- Sparse purpuric rash (Fig. 150).

Investigations

CSF smear, culture, glucose and protein (lumbar puncture); blood picture, glucose and culture.

Management

High dose antimicrobials for bacterial meningitis.

Prevention

Immunization against Hib. Rifampicin prophylaxis for contacts of *N. meningitidis* and *H. influenzae* infections.

Bell's palsy

Aetiology

Unknown—probably viral.

Pathology

Inflammation of the facial nerve.

Clinical features

Acute unilateral lower motor neurone facial palsy (Fig. 151).

Diagnosis

Clinical. Exclude chronic suppurative otitis media, temporal bone lesion, diabetes, hypertension, HIV and Lyme disease (*Borrelia burgdorferi* infection).

Management

- Protect eye (glasses/pad/artificial tears) (Fig. 152, p. 118).
- Immediate systemic prednisolone and aciclovir (though most recover spontaneously).

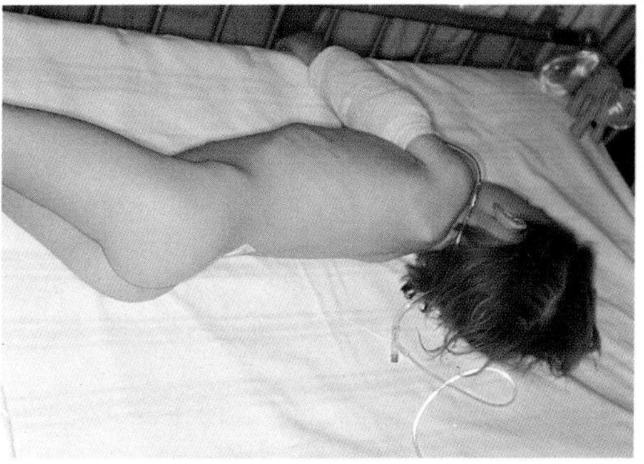

Fig. 149 Neck retraction and arched back in meningitis.

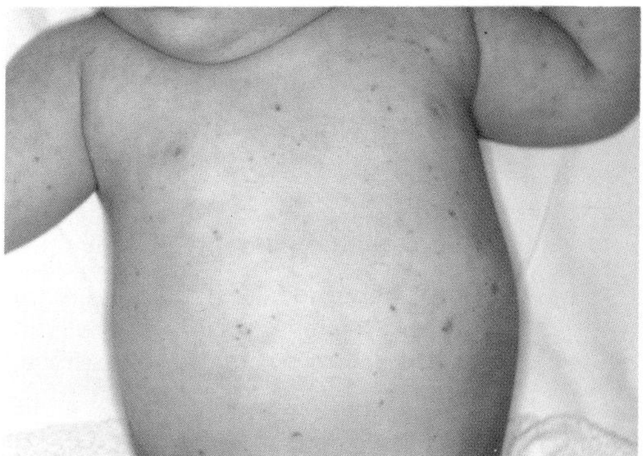

Fig. 150 Sparse purpuric rash typical of meningococcal septicaemia.

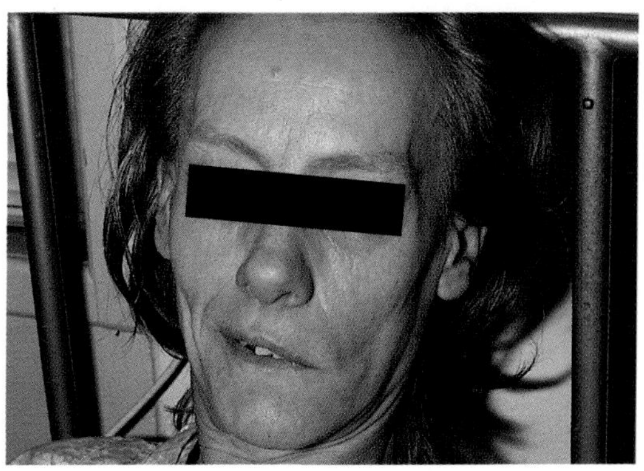

Fig. 151 Lower motor neurone facial palsy (Bell's palsy).

Motor neurone disease (motoneurone disease)

Aetiology

Idiopathic degeneration of motor neurones.

Pathology

Affects upper and lower motor neurones—never cranial nerves III, IV or VI (hence eyes move normally).

Clinical features

- *Amyotrophic lateral sclerosis* (50%)—flaccid arms and spastic legs.
- *Bulbar palsy* (25%) (see below).
- *Progressive muscular atrophy* (25%)—affects anterior horn cells, causing distal then proximal muscle atrophy (Fig. 153).
- *Primary lateral sclerosis*—rare.

Investigations

Electromyography (EMG) (to show denervation potentials) is occasionally useful.

Prognosis

Average survival is only 3 years.

Bulbar palsy

Aetiology

Motor neurone disease, poliomyelitis, Guillain–Barré syndrome (allergic polyneuritis).

Pathology

Lower motor neurone lesion affecting bulbar cranial nerves which supply muscles of tongue, mastication, swallowing and facial expression (Fig. 154).

Clinical features

- Tongue—weak, wasted and fasciculates.
- Speech—quiet, nasal or hoarse.
- Soft palate—weak.
- Swallowing difficulties.

Pseudobulbar palsy

Aetiology

Most commonly due to bilateral internal capsule lesions. It may also result from CVA.

Clinical features

- Tongue—spastic without wasting.
- Jaw jerk—increased.
- Speech—like Donald Duck.
- Emotions—labile.
- Swallowing difficulties.

Management

Physiotherapy and nursing.

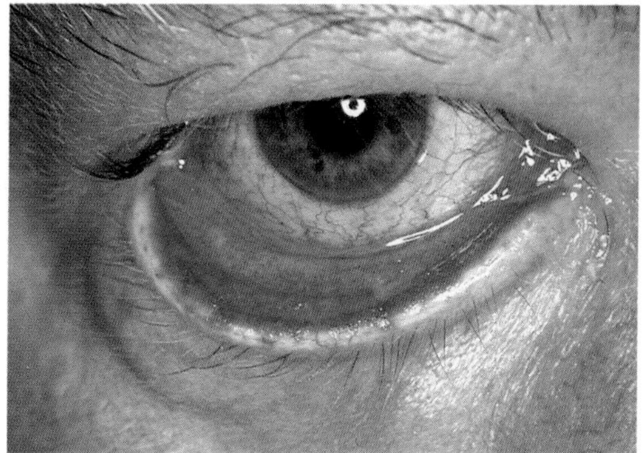

Fig. 152 Conjunctivitis secondary to facial palsy.

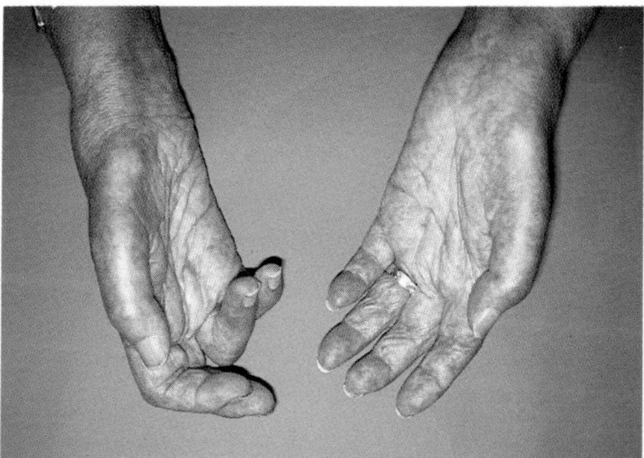

Fig. 153 Distal muscle wasting in motor neurone disease.

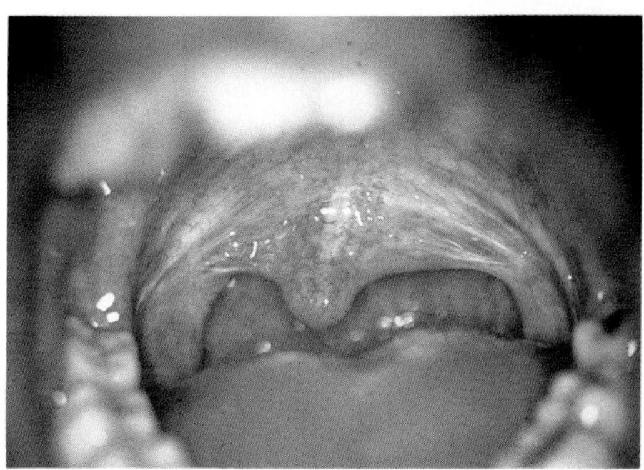

Fig. 154 Weakness of left vagus in bulbar palsy.

Myasthenia gravis

Aetiology Antibodies against acetylcholine receptors.

Clinical features Weakness after exercise and towards end of day. Initially the weakness is mainly of extraocular (e.g. ptosis), bulbar ('hanging jaw' sign) and neck muscles. There may be other autoimmune disorders or thymoma.

Investigations Anticholinesterase (edrophonium) improves symptoms.

Management Anticholinesterases; sometimes corticosteroids, thymectomy or plasmapheresis.

Duchenne muscular dystrophy

Aetiology X-linked recessive degenerative disease of muscles.

Clinical features Difficulty in walking, waddling gait, lumbar lordosis and difficulty in climbing stairs. The pectoral girdle is affected initially (winging of scapulae) (Fig. 155), and then the pelvic girdle (Fig. 156).

Prognosis Most are chair-bound by time of puberty.

Management Physiotherapy.

Cerebral palsy

Aetiology CNS motor damage in utero, at birth or postnatal.

Clinical features

- *Spastic* (70%)—hypertonia (hemiparesis). Both sides may be affected (quadraplegia) (Fig. 157) or lower limbs only (diplegia).
- *Dyskinetic* (10%)—involuntary movements of most muscles.
- *Ataxic* (10%)—hypotonia, weakness, incoordination and tremor.
- *Mixed* (10%).

There may also be learning disability, epilepsy and defects of special senses.

Management Special schooling, physiotherapy.

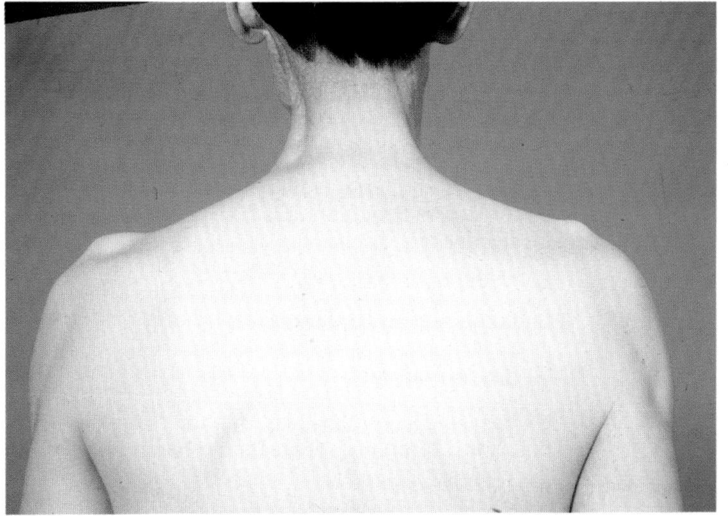

Fig. 155 Duchenne muscular dystrophy: gross wasting of the left trapezius muscle.

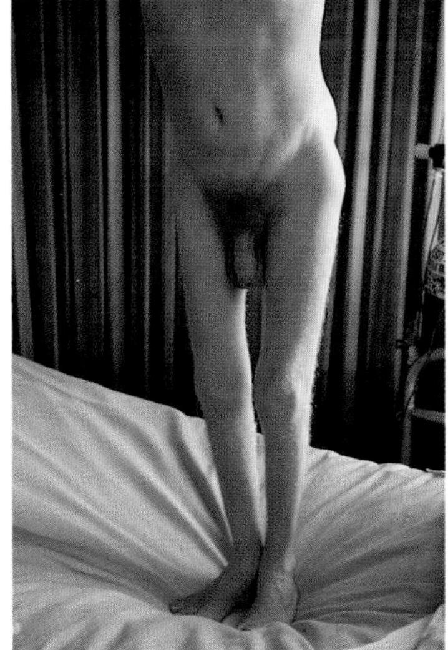

Fig. 156 Muscular dystrophy.

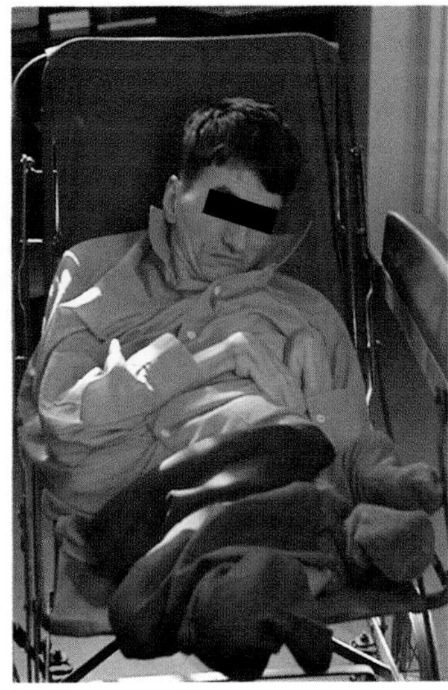

Fig. 157 Cerebral palsy.

CNS tumours

Pathology Most are metastases (e.g. from lung, breast). Primary neoplasms are gliomas (e.g. astrocytoma or oligodendroglioma). 30% are histologically benign (meningioma or neurofibroma).

Clinical features Headache, vomiting, papilloedema and later seizures. The condition may also produce other local signs (Fig. 158).

Investigations CT/MRI; possible biopsy.

Management Radiotherapy and/or surgery.

Hydrocephalus

Aetiology Decreased CSF outflow, e.g. due to congenital deformity, tumours, subarachnoid haemorrhage.

Clinical features Rapid enlargement of the cranium in children (Fig. 159). In adults there is headache, vomiting, papilloedema, ataxia and motor anomalies.

Management Shunting of CSF (ventriculo–atrial shunt).

Down syndrome (mongolism)

Aetiology 95% have trisomy 21. There is an association with advanced maternal age.

Clinical features Learning disability. Abnormal facies—flat face, epicanthic folds, brachycephaly (Fig. 160). Short stature and short neck. Broad hands with short fingers (brachydactyly) and simian palmar creases. Congenital heart defects. Gut defects. Liability to infection and acute leukaemia.

Diagnosis Prenatal amniocentesis or chorionic villous sampling.

Prevention Genetic counselling.

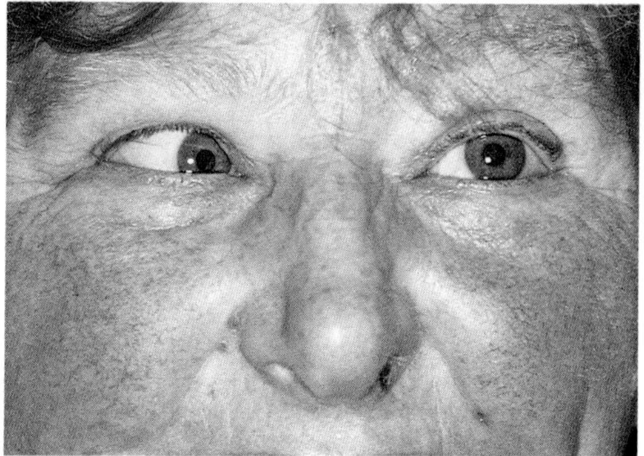

Fig. 158 Palsy of left abducens nerve: patient looking to her left.

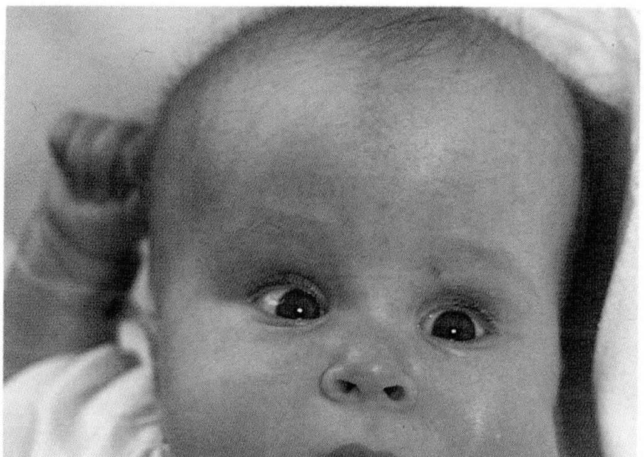

Fig. 159 Hydrocephalus: note 'sunset' eyes.

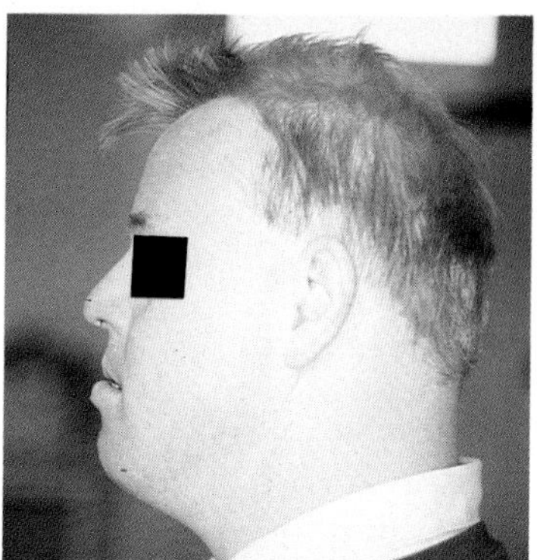

Fig. 160 Typical facies of Down syndrome.

13 / Rheumatic disease

Lupus erythematosus

There are systemic (SLE) and localized or discoid (DLE) forms of lupus.

Aetiology

Unknown—possibly viral; associated with genetic background.

Pathology

Autoimmune disorder (connective tissue disease).

Clinical features of SLE

- *Non-specific:* malaise, fever, depression.
- *Skin:* butterfly rash over nose/malar region (Fig. 161), Raynaud's phenomenon, purpura, alopecia.
- *Musculoskeletal:* myalgia, arthralgia.
- *Cardiopulmonary:* pericarditis, pleurisy.
- *Renal:* nephritis.
- *CNS:* various.
- *Haematological:* anaemia, thrombocytopenia, leucopenia.
- *Gastrointestinal:* anorexia, nausea, Sjögren syndrome.

Investigations

Antinuclear antibodies (ANA), antibodies to double-stranded DNA, immune complexes, low complement, raised ESR, blood picture (anaemia, perhaps neutropenia).

Management

Immunosuppressives in severe SLE; antimalarials in mild SLE.

Sjögren syndrome (SS)

Definition

Autoimmune exocrinopathy. Primary SS (SS-1) is dry eyes and mouth; secondary SS (SS-2) is when there is also a connective tissue disease.

Clinical features

Dry eyes (with or without lacrimal swelling), and dry mouth (with or without salivary swelling), glossitis and candidosis (Fig. 162). There may also be connective tissue disease and/or Raynaud's phenomenon.

Investigations

- Biopsy of salivary glands in lower lip.
- Autoantibodies (anti-Ro (SS-A) and anti-La (SS-B)) in serum.

Management

Artificial tears and saliva; sometimes pilocarpine.

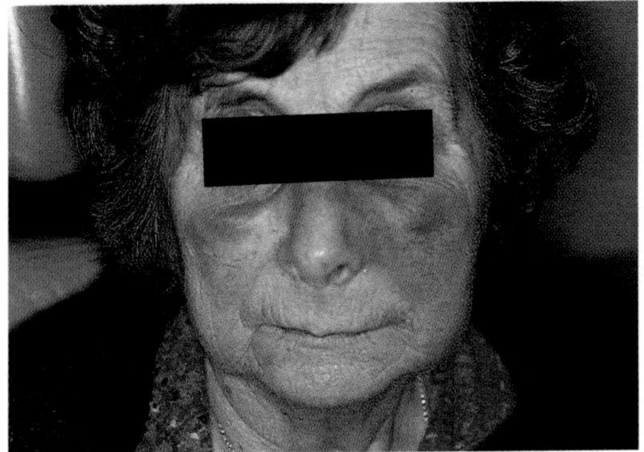

Fig. 161 Facial rash in systemic lupus erythematosus.

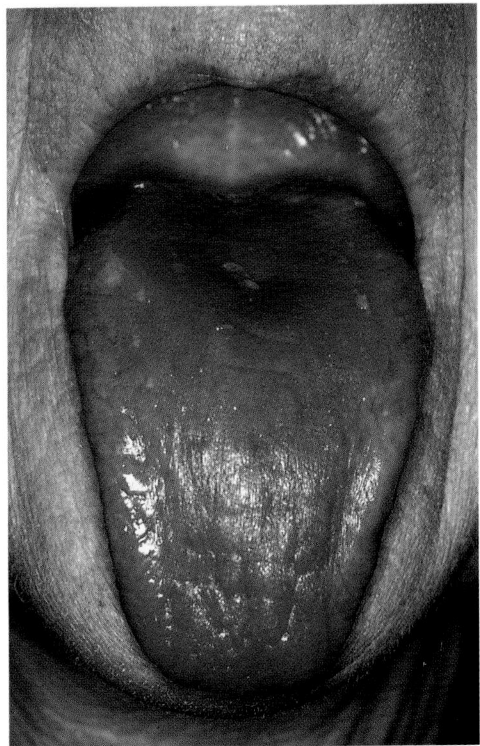

Fig. 162 Glossitis and candidosis in Sjögren syndrome.

Systemic sclerosis (scleroderma)

Aetiology

Unknown—probably immunological.

Pathology

Skin oedema followed by fibrosis, atrophy and loss of elasticity.

Clinical features

- *Skin*—taut, inelastic (Fig. 163), mucocutaneous telangiectasia. Raynaud's phenomenon in 75% (Fig. 164).
- *Others*—pulmonary fibrosis in 50%, oesophageal hypomotility in 80%, with occasional Sjögren syndrome renal, cardiac, hepatic or neurologic involvement.

Investigations

- Nuclear, Scl-70, or centromere autoantibodies.
- *Blood*—normocytic, normochromic anaemia.
- *Radiographs*—calcium deposits in fingers and eroded distal phalanges in some.

Management

Penicillamine, immunosuppressives or plasma exchange.

Amyloidosis

Aetiology and pathology

Idiopathic (primary) or usually secondary to chronic infections, inflammatory disorders, myelomatosis or haemodialysis. Extracellular deposits of abnormal protein stain with congo red or thioflavin T on histology.

Clinical features

- *Renal* (in over 75%)—proteinuria and haematuria; hypertension.
- *Cardiac* (in 30%)—ECG changes; cardiomyopathy.
- *Respiratory, gastrointestinal and skin*—amyloid deposits (Fig. 165); petechiae (Fig. 166).

Investigations

Biopsy of affected tissue, rectum or gingiva.

Management

- Manage underlying cause.
- Cytotoxics for plasma cell dyscrasia or systemic amyloid.
- Dimethyl sulphoxide (DMSO) may cause transient improvement.

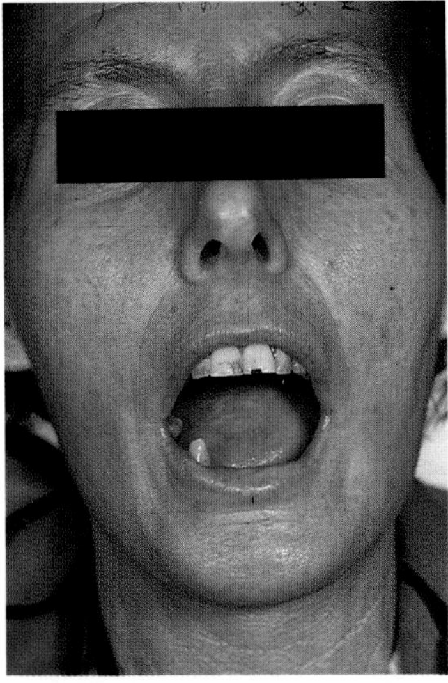

Fig. 163 Limited mouth opening and tight skin in systemic sclerosis, 'Mona Lisa' face.

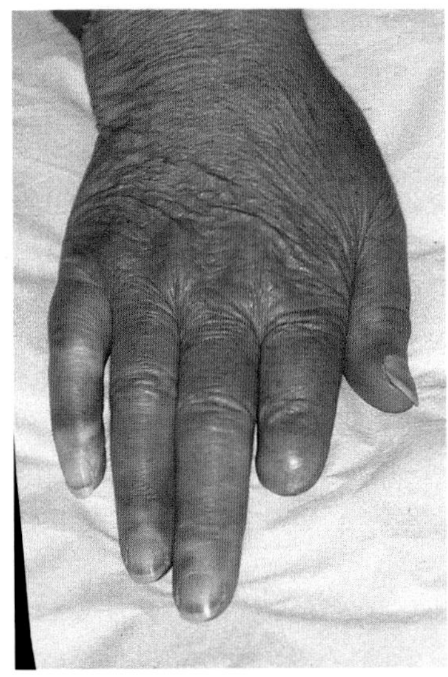

Fig. 164 Systemic sclerosis: loss of digit due to severe Raynaud's phenomenon.

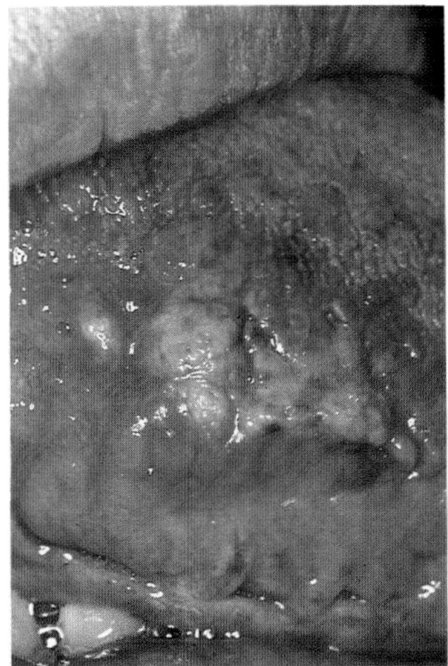

Fig. 165 Amyloidosis causing macroglossia.

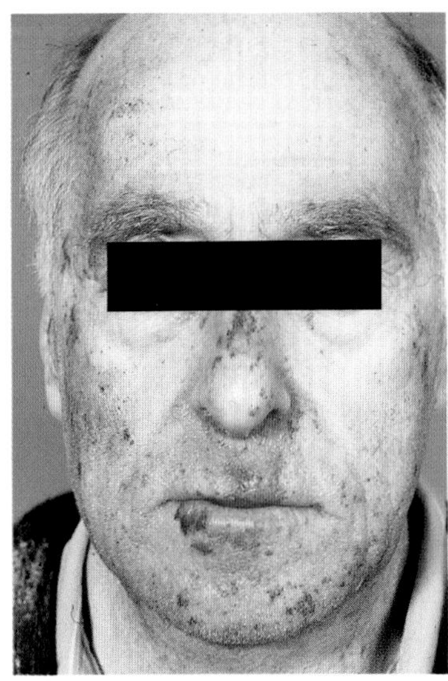

Fig. 166 Amyloidosis: petechiae due to bleeding tendency.

Rheumatoid arthritis (RA)

Aetiology

This connective tissue disease is possibly viral in origin in patients with a genetic predisposition.

Pathology

Mononuclear cell destruction of synovia. Immune complexes induce vasculitis.

Clinical features

Painful, swollen, stiff joints of mainly hands and feet. There is swelling and tenderness at the metacarpophalangeal (MCP) and *proximal* interphalangeal joints. Later developments are ulnar deviation, subluxation (Fig. 167) and dislocation at the MCP joints, and thumb and finger deformities with wasting of small muscles. The feet are similarly affected. Other regions may be involved (Fig. 168). May be Sjögren syndrome.

Investigations

- 75% have rheumatoid factor (RF); 30% have anti-nuclear antibodies (ANA).
- ESR—raised.
- Anaemias.
- Radiography—erosion of joint surfaces, loss of joint space, osteoporosis and bone cysts.

Management

Physiotherapy; non-steroidal anti-inflammatory agents; immunosuppression; surgery.

Osteoarthritis (OA)

Aetiology

Unknown.

Pathology

Erosion and splitting of cartilage.

Clinical features

Affects mainly the first MCP and metatarsophalangeal joints, and the *distal* interphalangeal joints of the hands. Hip, knee and C5–C7 and L3–L5 apophyseal joints may also be affected. Pain, and swelling of the distal interphalangeal joints (Heberden's nodes, Fig. 169) and sometimes of the proximal interphalangeal joints (Bouchard's nodes) are typical of the condition.

Investigations

Radiography—reduced joint space, and subchondral bone sclerosis, osteophytes and bone cysts.

Management

Analgesia, physiotherapy and, increasingly, surgery.

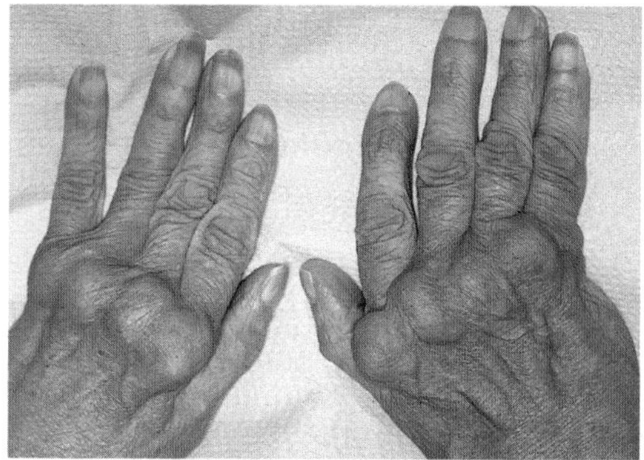

Fig. 167 Ulnar deviation and subluxation of joints in rheumatoid arthritis.

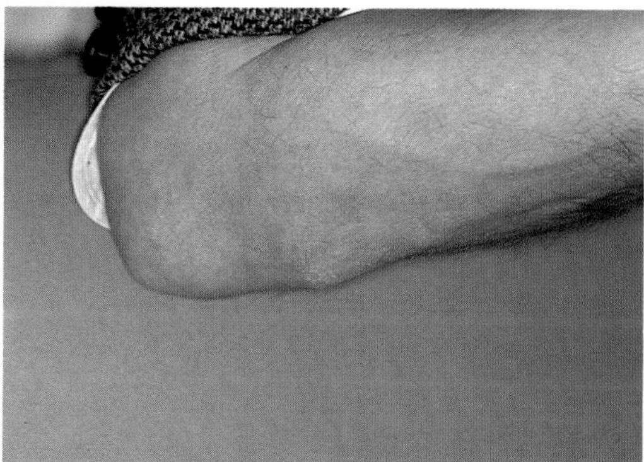

Fig. 168 Rheumatoid arthritis: subcutaneous nodules.

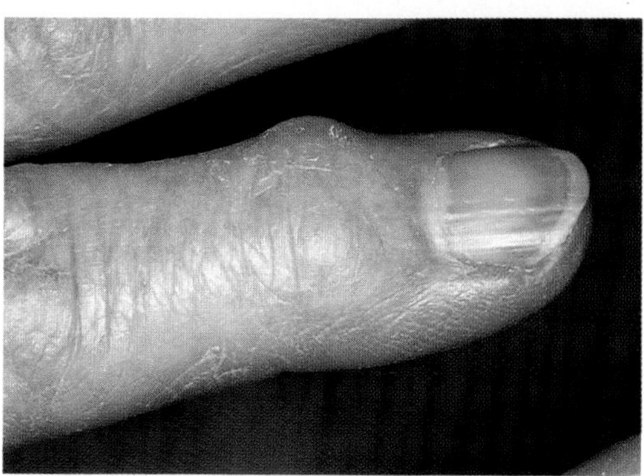

Fig. 169 Heberden's nodes in osteoarthritis.

Ankylosing spondylosis (spondylitis)

Aetiology Idiopathic; 95% have HLA-B27.

Pathology Sacroiliitis and ossification of vertebral interspinous ligaments.

Clinical features Pain and morning stiffness. Progressive ankylosis causes kyphosis and stooped posture (Fig. 170).

Investigations ESR; radiography—juxta-articular sclerosis, erosions and narrowing of sacroiliac joints, 'bamboo spine' (Fig. 171).

Management Exercise and physiotherapy; analgesia.

Reiter syndrome

Aetiology Gastrointestinal *Shigella, Yersinia, Salmonella* or *Campylobacter* infection, or non-specific urethritis; seen usually in HLA-B27 positive males.

Clinical features *Urethritis, conjunctivitis* and *arthritis* (Fig. 172), sometimes accompanied by low fever, oral ulcers, keratoderma blenorrhagica, balanitis or uveitis.

Investigations ESR may be raised. No specific investigations.

Management Non-steroidal anti-inflammatory agents.

Osteoporosis

Aetiology Associated with old age and the menopause. The disorder occasionally follows endocrine disease, immobilization, chronic renal failure or corticosteroids.

Clinical features Bone pain and liability to fracture and vertebral collapse (Fig. 173).

Investigations Plain radiographs may be helpful.

Management High calcium intake, hormone replacement, exercise.

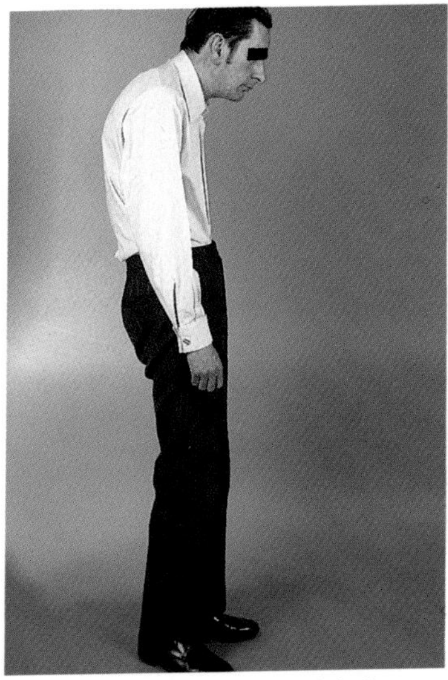

Fig. 170 Kyphosis (stoop) of ankylosing spondylitis.

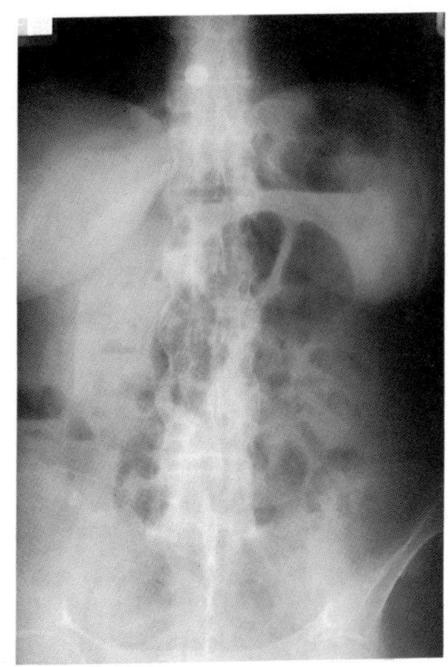

Fig. 171 Bamboo spine in ankylosing spondylitis.

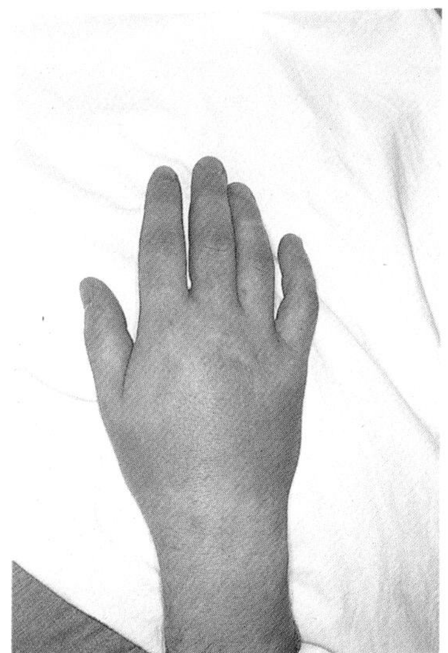

Fig. 172 Swollen hand due to arthritis in Reiter's disease.

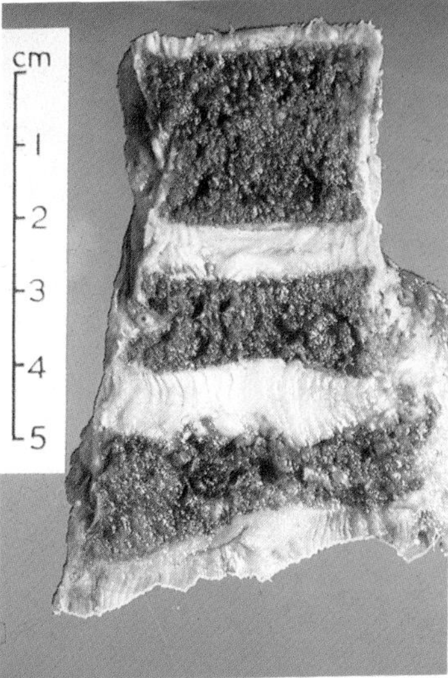

Fig. 173 Postmortem specimen of osteoporotic vertebral collapse.

Gout

Aetiology

Hyperuricaemia due to increased production (e.g. in myeloproliferative disorders) or decreased excretion (e.g. in renal disease), but usually idiopathic.

Pathology

Uric acid crystals in tissues (tophi, Fig. 174), joints or urinary tract (stones).

Clinical features

Acute episodes of pain, usually in the metacarpophalangeal joint of the big toe, later becoming chronic with tophi about joints. The hands are also often affected (Fig. 175). The condition is often precipitated by starvation, alcohol, drugs or surgery.

Investigations

Hyperuricaemia. Uric acid crystals in joint aspirate.

Management

Acute episodes:
- Non-steroidal anti-inflammatory drugs
- Aspirate joints and inject corticosteroid.

Prophylaxis: allopurinol.

Paget's disease of bone

Aetiology/ Pathology

Unknown cause. Excessive osteoclastic resorption with compensatory disorganized new bone formation.

Clinical features

- Bone pain and thickening.
- Bending of weight-bearing bones, e.g. femur, tibia (Fig. 176).
- Less commonly—nerve compression, arteriovenous shunting and osteogenic sarcoma.

Investigations

Radiology (thickened bones, cotton-wool radio-opacities, occasional radiolucencies, especially in the skull (Fig. 177, p. 134)). Bone scan (uptake increased). Serum alkaline phosphatase (increased). Increased urinary hydroxyproline. Biopsy, sometimes.

Management

Analgesics; calcitonin/sodium etidronate.

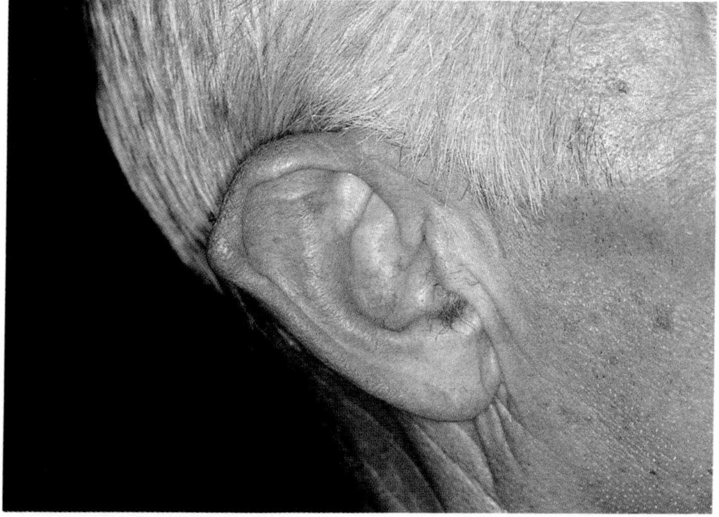

Fig. 174 Gouty tophus of the auricle.

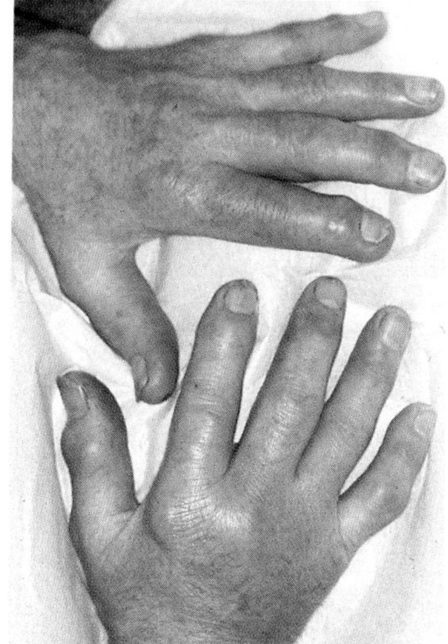

Fig. 175 Gouty arthritis of the hand.

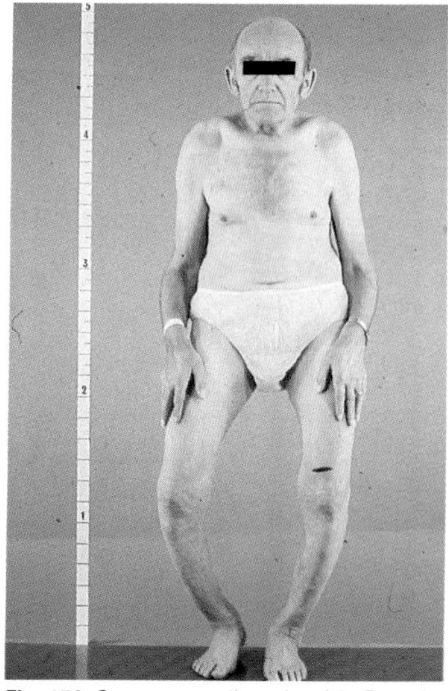

Fig. 176 Genu varum (bow legs) in Paget's disease.

14 / Diseases of the ear, nose and throat

Otitis externa

Aetiology Bacteria (e.g. *Staph. aureus, E. coli* or *Pseudomonas* spp.), *C. albicans* or *Aspergillus niger* introduced by trauma or poor hygiene.

Clinical features Pain, irritation, discharge and hearing loss (if canal completely occluded) (Figs 178 & 179).

Management Clean ear; analgesics; antibiotic and corticosteroid combination preparations; no swimming.

Acute otitis media

Aetiology Bacterial infection (e.g. *Strep. pneumoniae, H. influenzae*).

Clinical features Earache and deafness, with red bulging ear drum that may perforate and discharge.

Management Analgesia, antibiotics and sometimes drainage (e.g. myringotomy). Grommets are fitted to drain chronic secretory otitis media.

Acute tonsillitis

Aetiology Viral or bacterial (*Strep. pyogenes*) infection.

Clinical features Sore throat, dysphagia, earache, headache, malaise, pyrexia, cervical lymphadenitis, enlarged red tonsils.

Management Fluids; analgesia; antibiotics.

Complications Quinsy (peritonsillar abscess)—requires incision for drainage, analgesics, and/or high dose antibiotics.

Epistaxis

Aetiology Bleeding from nose due to respiratory infections, trauma, allergy, hypertension, bleeding disorders or other causes.

Management Cautery if bleeding point visible. Nasal packs or arterial ligation if uncontrollable.

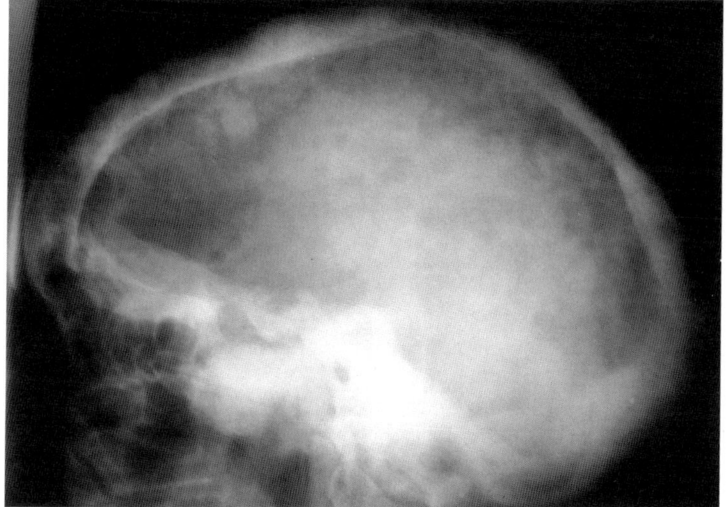

Fig. 177 Paget's disease of the skull.

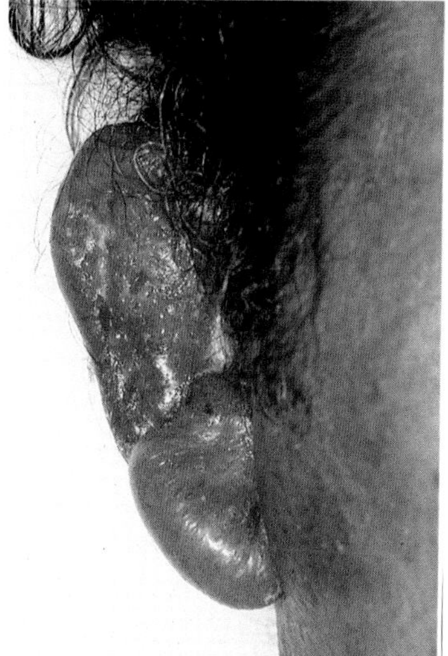

Fig. 178 Otitis externa.

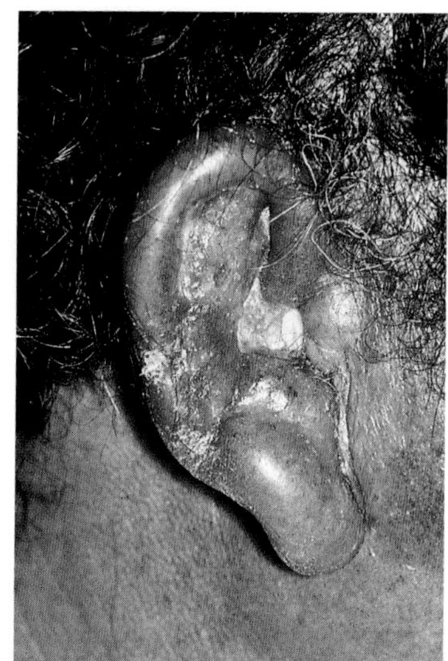

Fig. 179 Otitis externa due to sensitivity to local medicaments.

15 / Ocular disease

Strabismus (squint)

Aetiology

Non-paralytic (concomitant) squints: idiopathic or due to CNS damage.

Paralytic (incomitant) squints: caused by neuromuscular disease or trauma (Fig. 158, p. 122).

Clinical features

- Non-paralytic—eyes maintain the same angle of squint in all directions (Fig. 180).
- Paralytic—defect only obvious when eye attempts to move in direction of the affected muscle.

Management

- Non-paralytic—eye patch, eye exercises, glasses, surgery.
- Paralytic—surgery.

Light-near disassociation

Definition

Altered pupillary responses to light, yet intact accommodation reactions.

Aetiology

Adie's tonic pupil: denervation of ciliary ganglion which is usually unilateral. The pupil is moderately dilated, constricts slowly to light and tends to overconstrict slowly with near vision.

Horner syndrome: defective sympathetic innervation to eye which can be due to lesions from the CNS outwards. There can also be ptosis, enophthalmos and loss of facial sweating (anhidrosis).

III nerve palsies: for example, as a result of trauma.

Parinaud's dorsal midbrain syndrome

Clinical features

Pupil dilates to light (both direct and consensual) yet constricts with accommodation.

Management

Treat underlying cause.

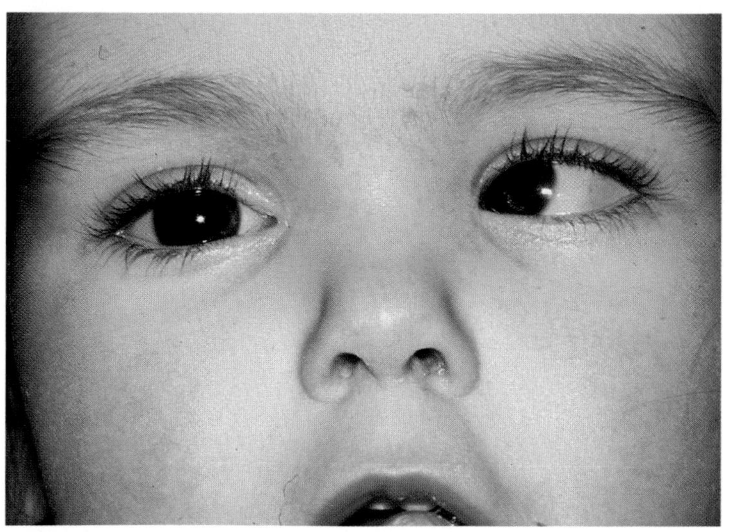

Fig. 180 Notable strabismus (squint). (The blue sclerae are normal in young children.)

Conjunctivitis

Aetiology
Upper respiratory virus or bacterial infection (*Strep. pneumoniae, Staph aureus*); trauma.

Clinical features
Conjunctival itchiness; swelling and erythema; epiphora (Fig. 181).

Investigations
Microbiological swabs.

Management
Usually chloramphenicol eye drops.

Uveitis (iritis)

Aetiology
Inflammatory disorders, e.g. TB, sarcoid, Behçet's disease, inflammatory bowel disease.

Clinical features
Painful red eye, blurred vision, photophobia, irregular pupil, pus in anterior chamber (hypopyon). The conjunctivae are normal.

Management
Systemic corticosteroids.

Keratitis

Aetiology
Viruses, staphylococcus, *Strep. pneumoniae*, trauma.

Clinical features
Painful watery eye.

Investigations
Slit lamp examination; swabs.

Treatment
Chloramphenicol drops, eye patch; aciclovir for HSV and VZV.

Cataract

Definition
Lens opacification.

Aetiology
Foreign bodies, trauma, diabetes, old age, intrauterine infection (e.g. CMV, rubella, toxoplasmosis, syphilis), drugs (e.g. corticosteroids), irradiation including ultraviolet and other causes.

Clinical features
Opaque lens, yellowing of visual image, loss of visual acuity, strabismus.

Management
Removal and replacement of lens.

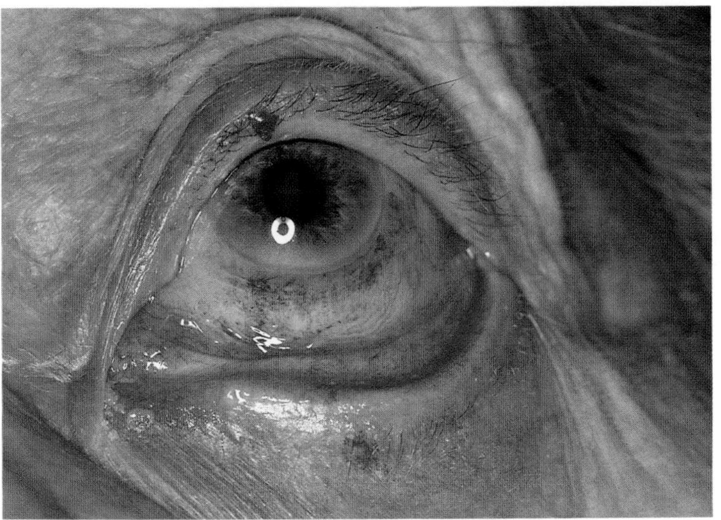

Fig. 181 Mild conjunctivitis in facial palsy. (The whitish line around the iris is an arcus senilis, an unrelated feature sometimes seen in old age.)

Index